Stem Cells for Osteoarthritis

ISBN: 978-1-963592-07-8
ISBN: 978-1-963592-08-5
ISBN: 978-1-963592-09-2

Published by Will Bozeman

For more information:
http://www.willbozeman.com

Table of Contents

WILL BOZEMAN

Willbozeman.com

Will@willbozeman.com

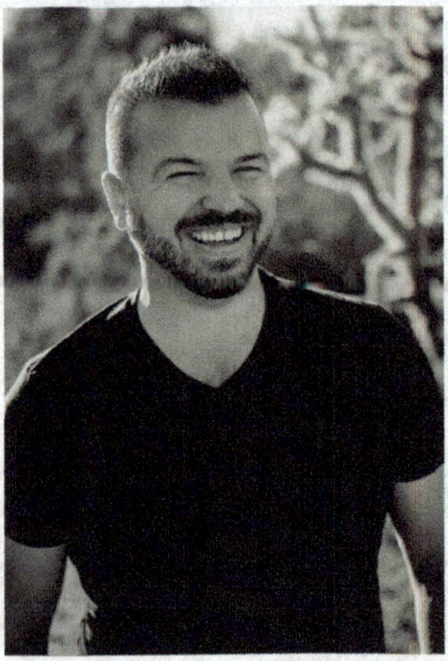

Will is a healthcare executive, innovator, entrepreneur, inventor, and writer with a wide range of experience in the medical field. Will has multiple degrees in a wide range of subjects that give depth to his capability as an entrepreneur and capacity to operate as an innovative healthcare executive. Will has an associate degree in electrical technology, two undergraduate degrees in biotechnology and archaeology, an MBA, and attended medical school in Alabama.

Will took a leave of absence from medical school to open his first biotech lab and serve as the chief science officer, writer, and innovator. Will has founded and launched multiple biotech ventures while serving in a range of positions in that field as chief executive officer, chief science officer, chief medical officer, founder, and innovator. Will has brought multiple biologic products to market for clinical use applications and written many treatment protocols for application of use and helped pioneer the use of regenerative medicine in the medical field.

If you've already read one of my stem cell books, you'll notice the first two chapters are the same. Just skip to chapter 3 if you want to jump straight into the main topic! Though, a refresher on the first two chapters never hurt anyone either.

Prologue

What an exciting age of medicine we live in today!

Stem cells and stem cell applications are already one of the greatest discoveries of modern medicine, and the vast majority of our advanced stem cell medical applications and uses are yet to come.

At the time of writing, there are countless studies on the clinical and medical application of stem cells from very specific disease conditions like specific cancers and congenital diseases, to more general use stem cell treatments for systemic inflammation, anti-aging and longevity, and even for use in aesthetic treatments like high-end facials and skin rejuvenation and hair regrowth.

Of course, some of the really interesting applications that researchers have their eyes on these days are advancements in nerve tissue regeneration and organ tissue growth and development.

I, for one, am excited for the day when we can simply grow organs for replacement instead of having a transplant list. Also, how about treating a range of chronic illnesses with a simple IV stem cell application on a regular basis?

There is no shortage of potential applications for use. However, for the purposes of this book I want to zero in on what is happening and available right now, what is available to patients in the United States, and what is available at the international stem cell treatment level.

My background and history in regenerative medicine

My background in stem cell biotechnology began with my biotech undergraduate degree, where I performed a range of cellular biotech functions, culturing and expanding various cell lines, isolating cellular DNA, and I conducted a range of lab testing procedures to prepare us for the exciting world of cellular biotech.

One of my favorite undergraduate projects that really helped me understand the details of the science of cellular biotechnology was to build a new cell culture lab for our university biotech department. This project really opened my eyes to how a cell culture lab worked and operated from start to finish. I didn't just learn how to do only specific tasks, like most students; I learned how everything worked, and the how and why behind it. I learned all about the current state of the industry because I had to build the lab. I had to order and test equipment; determine capabilities and functional uses; troubleshoot lab problems, operations and activity flow of the lab; determine the capabilities of what could be produced in a cell culture lab; and, of course, understand where the industry needed innovation and what was on the horizon.

Most students only got a tiny window into this world, but I was able to stand in front of a huge bay window and see what cellular biotech was all about. This is what really helped me understand the foundation of the world of regenerative medicine and started me down the path of stem cell therapy and regenerative medical applications.

Biotechnology is a notoriously risky field to be in because the people who are often exceptional with the science are not often exceptional with the business and practical applications. Luckily, I snagged my MBA before I went to medical school, so I have a little more understanding of the business of a biotech operation and how to make it succeed. It doesn't matter how lofty or noble your biotech ambitions are, if you can't pay your bills, you can't do anything to further your efforts … and people don't seem to like working for free.

Business and biotech are highly intertwined. Because there are so many variables to account for, biotechnology remains one of the more difficult categories of business to engage in, and yet it continues to attract hundreds and even thousands of new startups and ventures every year. I believe this is because of the allure of the magnitude of what can be accomplished or what could be developed if your idea succeeds.

The potential upside for success is more enticing than the risk/fear of failure. I've felt this strange dynamic many times. I'm looking at a potentially life-saving therapy and I can immediately convince myself that I would sacrifice my own financial security to get this treatment to market! I tell you this because this new era of amazing medical therapy is brought to you by innovators and pioneers in this field who often ride the edge of success all the way to the end, good or bad.

Particularly in the world of stem cells, the people I meet are not just thinking of how to start a business or get a good job, they are thinking of how to change the world. The potential for stem cell therapy to revolutionize many categories of medicine is very strong, and this is what drives everyone in this field.

I myself am guilty of diving headfirst into biotech startups because the potential benefits and applications are so exciting that I can't say no. To the surprise of my professors, I started my first lab company, stem cell processing, and storage lab while I was in my biotech undergrad program. It provided private processing and cryopreservation storage of cord blood and tissue for later stem cell therapies for parents who wanted that protection and assurance for their children.

My professors hadn't seen many students apply what they had learned so quickly in real life. I found myself in real-world conversations with professors over my company and the potential growth and expansion of my startup. I literally had conversations with my professors on the side of the classroom discussing investment and growth options while other students completed their regular course work. I tell you this because my undergrad experience was completely different from my peers.

This particular lab operation to process and store cord blood stem cells for parents having children who wanted to save those cells was more than just a business venture; I saw it as a calling, my first real life stem cell operation.

Cord blood stem cells provide a specific type of stem cell that could become valuable to a patient if they develop certain medical conditions down the road, but the only sure fire way to know you have a match available when you need it is to bank it yourself for later.

When I started this company, it was still very new in the market and the pushback was actually from the doctors in the hospital who didn't want to be bothered with having to collect the cord blood. Even though they usually aren't the ones doing it – it's almost always a nurse or medical assistant doing the actual collection – they still didn't like that it was a "new thing" to have to deal with.

I'll never forget the comment from the doctor who delivered our first child, regarding our collection of cord blood. "If we have time, we'll try to get to your science experiment." He referred to it as a frivolous science experiment and was annoyed that he had to be bothered with it. He was an older doctor and likely was not ready for this new world of advanced stem cell therapy.

A few years later I spoke to the partner in that same obstetrics office, and he said they had seen multiple children whose lives had been saved by cord blood banking and he was now an advocate for cord blood storage. His partner had mocked it only a few years before that, then suddenly it hit them that it's not just a science experiment, but an advanced lifesaving medical protocol. Suddenly, the world they work in is new and different, and people who previously would not be alive are now alive because of it. It happened that fast.

I continued that lab venture into medical school but had to hand it off to a colleague due to time constraints: med school is pretty busy. I was halfway through medical school when I was invited to co-venture and open a biotech lab focusing on stem cell processing and stem cell product manufacture for medical use by physicians in the orthopedic and pain management space. I took a leave of absence from medical school to be the chief science and medical officer for this biotech venture and opened this new biotech lab in Arizona, one of the hubs of biotech in the nation at that time.

I was already through the academics of medical school, and I realized two things pretty quickly. Firstly, what I was being taught was so far behind what I had already studied in biotech that if I wanted to be at the forefront of medical innovation, I would not get there by traditional medical school processes for at least a decade. Secondly, I could do so much more good in the medical world through my experience in biotechnology and business experience than I would finishing medical school and going into residency for several more years.

I saw the writing on the wall pretty quickly and chose the path of biotech and innovation. I'll forever be grateful for the medical knowledge I gained from my academic years in medical school; this education has greatly helped me in the process. I'll always advocate for education, but there's a point where you know what you know, you know what other people don't know, you know what you can do and what other people can't do or aren't doing, and you start seeing the opportunities where you can make a larger impact.

It took several months of contemplation to not go back and finish med school, but my path was already being structured for me through successful efforts in this new biotech venture I'd left med school for. I never looked back, and I have directly seen my positive impact at the national level in the field of regenerative medicine.

I built a tissue processing lab in Arizona and developed multiple product lines and lectured on stem cells and clinical applications at multiple medical conferences before my med school colleagues were finished with school.

As of the time of writing, I have started multiple biotech companies, multiple medical companies, built/owned/operated multiple clinical labs, developed dozens of products and services in the medical field, and written hundreds of pages of scientifically backed content for these operations and for product use in the medical field.

I have also written numerous treatment protocols for the application of regenerative medicine products in medical practice, and I've personally taught and coached hundreds of physicians and medical providers on the use and application of biologic products and many other aspects of the field of regenerative medicine, resulting in the direct application of therapy to tens of thousands of patients.

I would say that one of my greater achievements in this space has been the education, coaching, and awareness I've brought to hundreds of physicians around the nation. This has probably done more to advance regenerative medicine than anything else I could have done during those years after I left medical school.

I'm excited to bring this guidebook to you for personal education on your options for the various regenerative medicine treatments available in the United States and in the international medical field.

Let's dive in!

Chapter 1 – Stem Cells

Stem Cells 101

A stem cell is the foundation unit of cellular growth and development. It's basically a blank slate cell that can grow in any direction it needs for cellular development of the whole body.

The remarkable behavior of a stem cell is that when it divides into two cells, one cell will divert off into the type of cell it needs to become, and the remaining cell stays a stem cell and can split again and again to produce more and more cells as needed.

This process of a stem cell splitting into a new specialized type of cell is called differentiation, the process of becoming different. It's a nice scientific word for a stem cell changing into a different cell type, and you'll hear it a lot because it's the fundamental aspect of what makes stem cells so amazing; the secret sauce of why stem cells are so useful.

Stem cells differentiate over and over and over. This is where it really gets interesting. How long can this go on? How long can stem cells keep dividing and creating a new dedicated cell line while the original one stays a stem cell? Turns out, basically your whole life, though it slows down and there are DNA mechanisms for how long it can do this.

Telomeres are the ends of a DNA strand and are the most commonly discussed aspect of cellular replication because telomere length can determine how many times a cell can replicate. Telomeres don't code for things, but they make it possible for the rest of the DNA to work. This replication declining mechanism has been identified as, and believed to be, a source and ultimate cause of aging and age-related illnesses.

Simply put, telomeres measure our life span and capacity to age and die. As I mentioned before, a telomere is the extra end string of DNA left over after a cell has replicated its DNA. The easiest way to describe a telomere is this: you tie a shoestring, but you don't tie the knot at the very end, you tie it down where the strings meet the braid. You then have nice long strings left over. You need that long string in order to tie another knot, because you can't tie a good knot using a short string. Also, you still need a nice tight knot with no dangling strands, so you cut off the extra length of string hanging off that knot. That's how telomeres get shorter with each replication cycle.

Over time, each replication shaves a little DNA off the end of that string, so eventually there's no telomere string left to tie knots with. But you still need to tie those knots, so you start tying knots with actual DNA that codes for important things. That DNA is now being chopped off the ends as well, just like telomeres were before, and you start losing valuable DNA. This is the beginning of the end of that DNA strand. After a while, that shoe is barely hanging on and will most likely fall off with a little too much activity.

This simplified description helps explain how telomeres are associated with stem cell activity. The question of how long a stem cell can replicate is a bit more complex, but it's really easy to understand that there is a limit. Now you know two terms: differentiation and telomeres. You're on your way to being a stem cell expert!

The entire story of stem cells is a little more than I want to get into in this book, but what I do want to discuss is the category of stem cells that is currently applicable to medical use. These two basic concepts of differentiation and telomeres really summarize why we need stem cells in medicine. After a while you just aren't going to make enough cells fast enough to replace the aging/dying/damaged cells in your body and that is why everyone should be extremely excited about the new field of stem cell medicine.

You obviously want to learn about the tremendous advantages stem cell therapies have for average medical conditions. After all, this is a guidebook to stem cell therapy for a specific medical condition you're interested in learning about, so it makes sense that I get to brass tacks on this.

Stem Cell Types

Hematopoietic stem cells: (he-mat-o-poi-et-ic) Hematopoietic stem cells differentiate into blood-based cells. *Heme* is the medical scientific word for iron, and the medical word for anything to do with blood, because iron makes your blood red and transports oxygen.

For example, hematology is the study of blood, so that should help you remember that hematopoietic stem cells make your blood cells. Most stem cell therapies you'll hear about in the coming years are NOT hematopoietic based therapies, and that's why I wanted to mention them first and then put them aside while I get to the more popular and more diverse category of mesenchymal stem cells.

Mesenchymal stem cells: (mess-en-ky-mal) Mesenchymal stem cells differentiate into many other cell types. One of these types is musculoskeletal tissue, also known medically as MSK.

MSK tissue contains cells such as cartilage, bone, muscle, tendons, and connective tissues, which are of particular interest in regenerative medicine because there are so many conditions in this category that can be treated.

You need to remember the initialism MSK because this is what is used most of the time to describe this category. This means mesenchymal stem cells are the type that can regenerate tissues for all the various injuries we endure through the daily activities of life. Everything from tendonitis and osteoarthritis to serious spinal injuries would look to mesenchymal stem cells as a possible treatment.

In order to explain the treatment possibilities with mesenchymal stem cells, there are two more terms I want to teach you here: autologous and allogeneic. Autologous means it comes from you; allogeneic means it comes from someone else and is given to you. These two terms define the entire state of stem cell therapy in the US and internationally.

See, you are really becoming a stem cell expert because most people have no idea those two terms exist or what they mean, much less that those two terms are how the world of stem cell therapy is divided up.

What is and what is not an actual stem cell treatment?

Buckle in and I'll run through a snap account of the regenerative medicine product portfolio in the market today. I'll follow up after this on where you're likely to see and hear about these different products and therapies, what to look for, and what to avoid.

Stem Cell Treatments and Products

The first thing you have to know is that the term "stem cells" became a common vernacular term for any regenerative product because it was the preferred term to use. This is because it was such a high-end medical term and because there were so many different products, it was hard to explain the differences, so everyone just called everything stem cells. This caused a lot of confusion and, ultimately, got the attention of the FDA and the FTC; I'll explain those details later.

Here we go:

Bone marrow stem cells: (autologous) Bone marrow stem cells are collected from your own bone marrow, processed, refined and concentrated, and reinjected into the target treatment areas. This is considered the traditional standard stem cell treatment in the US, and this has been the gold standard for treating musculoskeletal conditions for the last couple of decades. There are pros and cons to this method but it's still the gold standard in the US for real and actual stem cell treatments for MSK conditions.

A wave of non-bone marrow frozen products came to market in recent years and has since declined and bone marrow is still the standard, proving that bone marrow stem cell treatments are still the gold standard of stem cell treatments for musculoskeletal conditions in the US.

The downside is that it requires a moderately uncomfortable procedure to collect bone marrow aspirate stem cells (BMAC), and the cells are technically as old as you are, so that whole section on telomeres now starts to make sense; your own stem cells are not any younger than you are.

However, the outcomes produced with bone marrow treatment from some of the leading medical groups using bone marrow stem cells show amazing results, and you can't argue with results. The leading groups can also prove that bone marrow stem cells ultimately save you and our healthcare system a LOT of money by using this treatment instead of a range of other conventional treatments and surgeries.

Ultimately, a really good bone marrow stem cell procedure can cost a fraction of the total cost of a major surgery, which would have been the conventional option. So, we're definitely on the right track in medicine with this procedure. Also, for your reference, you'll often hear bone marrow stem cells referred to as BMA or BMAC, which is bone marrow aspirate or bone marrow aspirate concentrate, respectively.

Adipose stem cells: Adipose stem cells are stem cells collected from your fat tissue through a liposuction procedure. These are becoming more popular for several reasons, but ultimately, it has been a battleground for regenerative medicine advocates because of legal issues and unscrupulous medical offices making claims of a wide range of cures. I am no expert on the latest in this legal and compliance battle but I read about it and hear about it often.

Remember, even a product that works can fail if the people using it make unsubstantiated claims, are abusive in their marketing tactics, or are abusive in pricing the treatment. Also, this requires liposuction to collect the fat and harvest the cells, so it's still invasive. Ultimately, it needs to be an available tool in the stem cell treatment category, so I'm hoping it continues its path to better compliance and standardization.

Cultured expanded stem cells: This is my favorite category of stem cell treatment because it's THE future of stem cell therapy worldwide.

Cultured and expanded stem cells are grown in specialized cell culture labs and can be grown using autologous or allogeneic stem cells. So you can use your bone marrow stem cells and grow them out to get a proper high dose for treatment, or you can use compliant perinatal tissue stem cells. You can isolate and grow a tremendous quantity of specific mesenchymal stem cells and have enough for multiple treatments all at the same time.

The ultimate problem with bone marrow or adipose cells is that you can only get so much material, so you can only create enough high dose stem cell content for limited use. Cell expansion is the future of stem cell treatment because you can grow just about as much as you need or want. Also, with advanced techniques, you can stimulate stem cells to differentiate into other cell types in the culture process.

Think: growing a batch of cardiac stem cells specifically for heart repair, or a batch of cartilage tissue stem cells for joint injuries! Also, think: lab grown organs and tissues. This is THE advantage in stem cell medicine and therapy and the future of cellular medicine as it becomes more formalized and standardized for predictable outcomes.

This is much more efficient than personal autologous collection methods like bone marrow or adipose collection procedures. The reason we see so much bone marrow and adipose activity in the US is because cultured expanded cells are prohibited in the US medical system. This is mostly for good reasons though, as it's very complicated to get it right and it needs to be refined and standardized for wide-scale application. Standardizing cellular therapy is not like other manufactured medications of treatments where chemistry can replicate the same molecule perfectly. Cell culture is like trying to encourage the cells to replicate the way you want, but you can't always count on it to be a perfect replication process. This is why it's hard to regulate cultured cell therapies, but the industry is getting much better at these processes.

I intend to be a part of the cellular therapy standardization process in the US because it's definitely the future of medicine, but I don't want it to be in a field that is bombarded with bad actors trying to game the market. As of this writing I am working with my team on some of these standardized cultured expanded stem cell therapies with plans and hopes to conduct trials and help get these treatments through the approval process in the US.

As luck would have it, several groups are already experts in cultured expanded cell therapies on the international level, so you can still get these procedures done today – just outside the US – and the applications are amazing! The range of conditions being treated with startling outcome s is very exciting. At any time while reading this book you can reach out to me and I'll direct you to some of the best options for this around the world.

Obviously, the MSK category is already a highly popular category, but now we are seeing movement into treatments for things like COPD (chronic obstructive pulmonary disease), heart tissue repair, neural tissue repair, eye and ocular healing and repair, advanced esthetics and hair regeneration, and, of course, one of my favorites, longevity and anti-aging therapies through full-body inflammation reduction via IV stem cell therapy.

There are a lot of other really exciting things, but I don't want to suggest that these conditions are being cured with these stem cell treatments yet. Some treatment types are helping these people and, in many cases, it's about the only available option that will work, even if it's a modest result. I personally knew a retired medical doctor who sought treatment for his chronic condition. I don't want to say what it was because I don't want to suggest that what he did will work for anyone else, nor that cultured expanded cell therapy will treat or cure this particular condition or act as a treatment option just yet, but he had very impressive results and I almost didn't believe it. Unfortunately this treatment only curbed the symptoms, which is still amazing for what it was able to do for him. The condition came back eventually, but the severity of his symptoms was significantly reduced and mostly resolved for nearly a year after that treatment. I can think of many people and many conditions where if there was a routine annual stem cell treatment that only reduced the severity of the symptoms, it would still be a tremendous success and would become the new standard of care for that condition. His results were something I didn't believe would happen at all. I knew the guy decently well; he was a retired family practice doctor. So our conversations on his treatment process were very interesting. He made me believe that what they are saying they're able to do in the international stem cell treatment market is actually possible using cultured expanded stem cell therapies.

I'll point you to some of these groups at the end of the book but want to make a disclaimer here. I know it's exciting, but it's still a very new field so I'm not suggesting or claiming that any condition I mention or discuss is curable or can be cured with these treatments … yet. I simply believe it is the right track to a better future of medical treatment.

Birth tissue stem cell products: Immediately, I want to point out that the birth tissue stem cell products I'm talking about here come from perfectly ethical and legally donated tissues that come from normal, healthy Cesarean section deliveries of donors who are fully informed about the procedure and go through rigorous and regulated vetting, screening, and testing. I know a lot about this process as I've launched multiple companies and labs that made these birth-tissue-based regenerative products. The best way to think of how this is compliant and moral and ethical is to understand that during a regular c-section delivery the mother and the baby are safe and healthy and they both move on with their life like normal, but what about all the leftover birth tissues involved in the process? Those tissues are normally disposed of as medical waste, but they are perfectly healthy tissues that can be repurposed into something useful. This is exactly what the perinatal birth tissue category has accomplished, using healthy safe tissues that are safely, ethically, and morally collected and processed into useful medical products. It's a wonderful way to make something useful out of something that would otherwise be useless.

All the collection programs I worked with in my career were heavily regulated by the FDA and a very detailed paper trail was in place for each tissue collection we received. I've explained the appropriateness of this category of tissue collection to hundreds of doctors and patients. Everyone is skeptical after hearing about some of the bad actors in the industry mentioned in news articles. I'd be skeptical, too, if I hadn't actually been in the middle of this process for so long. I've seen so much good come from this treatment category, and, of course, where there's good there's going to be a few bad actors exploiting that good, and I'll tell you about those as well later.

There is a range of products created from perinatal birth tissues. Two of the primary reasons birth tissues are so useful are: first, the cells are brand new, so they are young and active and have a full life cycle of replication potential, if you recall the topic of telomeres and stem cell replication lifespan.

The second reason is that the cells in the tissues have little to no detectable immunomarkers on the cells. This means that you don't have to type match a donor to a recipient like you do with blood and organs. I've explained this concept to several hundred doctors over my biotech career because, to the average trained physician, our cells have markers that identify ourselves versus foreign cells.

The short answer to why these tissues have little to no detectable immunomarkers is that the mother and the developing baby are two unique entities with their own identifying immunity markers. So if they could sense each other's presence, they'd fight each other with their own immune responses.

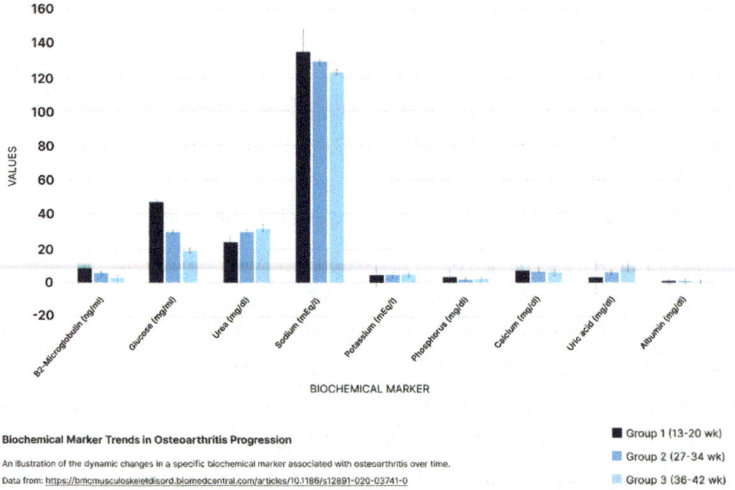

Biochemical Marker Trends in Osteoarthritis Progression

An illustration of the dynamic changes in a specific biochemical marker associated with osteoarthritis over time.

Data from: https://bmcmusculoskeletdisord.biomedcentral.com/articles/10.1186/s12891-020-03741-0

Birth tissues like the placenta, umbilical cord, and amniotic membrane are created specifically to overcome this problem by being immune marker neutral tissues. The amniotic fluid, membrane, umbilical cord, and placenta are designed to shield the two entities from each other, thus making the tissues ideal for use as a stem cell source because the cells won't have immune markers to trigger responses.

Here's a list of the different birth tissues that are popular for stem cell collection:

Industry note: At the time of writing, all birth tissue injectable biologics are being reclassified under FDA regulations, so you may not see many of these in the market anymore until regulators iron out how they will be allowed moving forward.

Amniotic fluid stem cells: This is the actual fluid that the fetus floated in and lived in during development. Naysayers love to claim this is just baby urine, but I've only ever heard this argument when a doctor is trying to sell you what they're offering that isn't amniotic fluid. Also, with all the studies on amniotic fluid in recent years, they've been proven wildly incorrect over the last decade for trying to suggest that amniotic fluid is mere baby urine. Again, they're only saying that if they're trying to sell you something else. Whether intentionally selling something else or unintentionally due to lack of education on the details, it's not the same world we lived in 20 years ago when it comes to understanding biologics.

Though it's true that babies do "urinate" a mild diluted version of urine in amniotic fluid, they also continuously drink amniotic fluid as well because it is completely safe for the fetus to consume, and this fluid is filled with high levels of, and a wide range of, growth factors and nutrients. It's nature's perfect regenerative fluid.

Remember that the baby's actual harmful waste is removed through the mother via the umbilical cord, not the baby, so all the harmful elements of urine waste have to be removed so they do not concentrate in the baby's liquid waste where it would build up to dangerous levels in amniotic fluid. So, if you hear "baby urine," then you know you're being sold, or the doctor isn't very solid on their regen med background.

However, I like to look at it as an opportunity to learn and grow. After all, I taught hundreds of doctors a wide range of regen med topics over the years that helped them apply therapies to patients. They have to start somewhere, and most of the time the doctors I taught were starting from scratch. I applaud them for leaping into the future!

Amniotic fluid comes in two main forms: fresh frozen and room temperature sterilized. I've worked with many versions of both and seen amazing outcomes with both for many years.

There may be a few viable stem cells in fresh amniotic fluid by the time it's injected into a patient, but nowhere near enough to justify calling it a stem cell injection, not to mention that many amniotic fluid products intentionally screen out the cell content. Also, when a doctor or medical office says their product has millions of stem cells, and they're located in the US, they're talking about general cell content, NOT stem cell counts.

What percentage of cells in these tissues are actual stem cells? It varies, but in amniotic fluid, for example, about 2-3% of the cell content is actual stem cells; the rest are all sorts of other tissue cells.

In the US we are not allowed refine and concentrate stem cells out of birth tissues into a concentrated injection, so if the doctor is taking a vial out of the freezer, you're not getting a vial full of stem cells, you're getting a vial full of a homogenous tissue composed of mostly non stem cells and tissue particulates, an injection with very few stem cells that most likely will not be viable living healthy cells by the time they are injected.

So, you can see how this is misleading if a medical office is advertising stem cell treatments and claims to have high quantities of stem cells in the injection. That's outright misleading and that's what has gotten the attention of the FDA and gotten the Federal Trade Commission, FTC, involved in regulating what doctors say to patients and what biotech labs and sales reps say to doctors.

Will's Industry Insight #1:
Ultimately, after 30,000+ cases using products created in my labs throughout my biotech career, the general consensus from the doctors and practices I've worked with is that fresh frozen amniotic fluid works better and produces better and longer outcomes.

Will's Industry Insight #2:
Genuine amniotic fluid is not considered a stem cell product, yet it has been routinely called stem cells as a common use vernacular term by doctors and pretty much everyone else in the industry. Now you can see how easy it is to confuse the different names of treatments and confuse patients on what they're getting.

Will's Industry Insight #3:
"Is my doctor selling me a certain number of cells?" If you're in the US then the short answer is no, not really, at least not really stem cells. Again, being a biotech founder, product developer and manufacturer, and working closely with hundreds of doctors gives you a lot of insight into how easy it is to misunderstand what the product is and how to describe it to a patient.

Despite the lack of genuine stem cell quantities in ready to go products in the US market, here's the real kicker you won't hear from your doctor or medical office: pure acellular amniotic fluid works as well as or better than cellular based injections ... without any cell content! You won't hear that from the office trying to sell you a treatment based on stem cell counts or stem cell viability content, but I've seen and heard this many times in offices that do a lot of treatment volume. This is what actually led me to create an acellular product line in the first place. Make a pure amniotic fluid product with no cell content. It worked tremendously well and outperformed a wide range of other products that claimed to have cell content.

As I mentioned before, if it's in the US and they're advertising an allogeneic stem cell product, aka a frozen, ready to go injection taken out of the freezer, with a specified cell count, they are not being honest with you about what you're buying, or the doctors themselves are not aware of what they are selling.

Either way, you're not getting what you think you're getting. Aside from that, the assumption for years was that the relatively few viable stem cells in the product are what produced the amazing outcomes everyone was seeing.

Despite the debate over cell content, most doctors I've worked with claim they see as good or better outcomes with pure fluid with no cell content. So, you can see that cells or no cells, it works. So it really does matter what the doctor is selling you and that you're aware of what you're paying for. But for your own peace of mind, that product you did get injected will probably work well and these nuances won't really matter. It just helps shape the background of the industry we are in to understand all these details.

Unfortunately, it's too easy to just call everything stem cells, but I believe once you attach a price to that stem cell quantity claim you're making, you have to be able to verify that claim, and doctors can't do that in the office, nor can the labs do that once it's in the doctor's office and out of the lab setting. Call it what it is and let the results speak for themselves, because the results are still great, they just need to get the messaging right.

I've been asked/recruited/petitioned vigorously by multiple labs and startups to help them create unique birth tissue products to take to market. They all want something they can call their own, something unique, something different, ultimately so they can corner the market on that one type of product that is unique to them.

It's not all bad for companies to want something special. It really is the driver of innovation and positive change in this industry. Because of this drive to innovate for novel products, we've landed on some amazing products in the market and the possibility that there will be FDA-approved products in coming years. It's all spurred by competition and drive to make something new.

Stem cells are such a new field, doctors don't get educated on it in medical school. I know because I asked about it specifically and my med school professors told me it wasn't a viable subject to teach yet because it was so new. While they were saying those words in class, I was actively developing the product manufacturing process for my first biotech product venture to isolate cell-rich tissues and make injectable products. We were seeing tremendous results with this product all while my professors wouldn't even acknowledge these as viable treatment options.

So where do the docs learn about it while in practice? Pretty much from the sales reps making rounds in their offices. Now I won't go into how risky this is, but I know exactly how these companies craft their products and messages to appear better, unique, different, and something extra special, and, in some cases, something that it actually isn't, as I've stated above.

Will's Industry Insight #4:
They all work about the same anyway! Most birth tissue products have roughly the same outcomes, despite what tissue they're derived from, or the cell counts or anything else. I've talked to many doctors about this, and they all agree that the outcome differences between one type and another are nominal, meaning the differences are nominal, but the outcomes are good across the board.

So … why the range of products? The ability to make a different product and stand out in the biotech market is a possibility for any biotech company, so it's attractive to create a unique product rather than just copy another. This was a very common practice for years and created the "wild west" of new biologic regenerative medicine products.

Will's Industry Insight #5:
Everything your doctor knows about stem cells, they've learned from a sales rep, or at least this was the norm for years and years. It's an unfortunate truth that the vast majority of what you're hearing in the doctor's office was taught by a sales rep for whatever product company is selling the product and it did not come from medical education or personal research by the doctor.

That said, I can tell in about five seconds if a doctor is reciting sales material education to me or if they know what they are talking about. I had my own set of questions I'd ask that would "prove out" the doctor as reciting sales rep info as their own knowledge. So I can say from experience that most of the doctors I've talked to, who endeavored to be in the regenerative medicine space, learned everything they know about it from sales reps. Don't even get me started on the sales reps and product distributors in the market. Most of the reps I've talked to couldn't speak to stem cells or regen med beyond what is printed on the brochure. Some of them are earnest and trying to do good and earn a living, others not so much. I used to indulge these reps when they wanted to sell me on their company's products, or try to recruit me to their company, and I've been the secret shopper for doctors trying to learn the details of a product and been on those phone calls or even in the office to hear the pitch and ask the "hard questions" that the rep should know if they know anything at all. Some of the doctors I've helped have connected with me for years to help them evaluate a new company or product, needing someone to make sense of the confusion in the market for them.

Will's Industry Insight #6:
"My chiropractor said 'stem cells' were reimbursed by Medicare." How many times have I heard this from patients? I stopped keeping count. Hundreds of doctors and chiropractors around the nation billed insurance and Medicare for "stem cell" products that were never reimbursable in the first place.

I've been on dozens of calls to explain why they couldn't do this and what the risk was going to be, and they preferred to believe the commissioned sales rep because what they were saying was more exciting … and profitable. So, no, currently you can't get your stem cells reimbursed by Medicare and the doctors and chiropractic offices who are telling patients this are incorrect.

Additionally, the risky part is that these are usually not professional sales reps like salaried employees who speak for the company, but commission-only sales reps who were never actually medically trained, have never operated professionally in the medical space or, in some cases, never went to college, and here they are "teaching" doctors about stem cell treatments because they have a brochure. That's why I push for doctors to do their own research and read their own white papers on the subject.

I could go into the specific details of why this wasn't allowed, but the short answer is that it's pretty clear in the reimbursement system that there is no reimbursement for unapproved biologics, and if you get reimbursement on it, those payers like Medicare and Commercial insurances can come take that money back from the medical office later after they figure out that the product and treatment wasn't covered.

Not necessarily a problem for patients to deal with, but it can destroy a medical office if they get all that reimbursement clawed back later, which I've seen many times. So it's just a matter of time. I've literally had dozens of calls with office and billing companies about the risk of them trying to bill for these products.

I actually pleaded with one doctor who was a friend of mine not to do this. He acted like he'd found this secret success in being able to bill insurances for these treatments. He didn't listen to me. He got clawed back by multiple insurances all at the same time and he had to shut down his office. It was sad, but I tried my best. Fortunately one of my other friends took my advance and avoided it. Then he called me a few months later to thank me for keeping him out of all that mess.

Will's Industry Insight #7:
"What's the deal with chiropractors selling stem cells?" Yep, I know it doesn't make sense at all, but I can explain. I'll add a disclaimer to this by saying not all chiropractors fall into this explanation category. Chiropractors are not medical providers, so they need to hire a medical provider to offer medical treatment in their offices.

Chiropractors are not medical physicians or medical providers, so they need to hire a medical provider to offer medical treatment in their offices. Years ago, chiropractors discovered that if they hired a genuine medical provider, such as a nurse practitioner (NP), physician assistant (PA), or an actual medical doctor (MD/DO), even just part-time for one day a week, they could effectively operate like a de facto medical office and offer genuine medical treatments instead of only chiropractic adjustments and related work.

In most states, medications, medical therapies, medical procedures, and medical treatments are outside the scope of a chiropractor's license. So, with a part-time medical provider on staff, a chiropractor can now offer all sorts of medical treatments for which they normally are prohibited from engaging in.

So, how did chiropractors get so heavy in the stem cell market when they aren't even allowed to prescribe that treatment or perform the injections? The short answer is that it was a new, high-end, medical procedure that actually worked well to relieve pain and, most importantly, it could be administered by a part-time medical provider who came into the office once a week to perform all the procedures that the chiropractor sold to their patients during the week.

With an NP who comes once or twice a week, you can offer all these treatments and schedule them all on the day the NP is on site and operate like a medical office in the eyes of the patient, and in many cases going the extra mile and removing chiropractic from the office name to enhance the medical aspect of the office. A chiropractic office that employs a medical provider is usually called an "integrated chiropractic office," or simply an "integrated office" for short. This model has been very common for the last couple of decades.

In fact, there are whole consulting companies dedicated specifically to coaching chiropractors to appear like medical offices in the market, using this term "integrated medical office," where the intent is to rename your practice to something that doesn't include the term chiropractor in the title. I've seen dozens of chiropractic offices change their names under these consultant groups' instructions. I've asked several of them why they changed the name and removed any reference to chiropractic services and the answers are that they want patients to see them as a genuine medical office with medical treatments, not just chiropractic services, even though the majority of the time the office is open there may not be a medical provider on site at all.

There's nothing wrong with a nurse practitioner working in a chiropractic office in this way, except when it becomes confusing to the patient about who is practicing medicine or who is the medical authority in the office. A chiropractor is not a medical authority over a genuine medical provider like an NP, PA, or MD/DO, so if a patient is confused about this, it creates problems, yet it's that state of confusion that many chiropractors have counted on in order to sell high dollar stem cell treatments for years. Many states are starting to look at this model because if the chiropractor pays the salary of the medical provider, then the medical provider may be incentivized to perform medical services under the direction of the chiropractor, which they are not allowed to do because medical therapies are outside the scope of a chiropractor, and chiropractors are not allowed to dictate the course of medical care to a medical provider.. You can see how this is also confusing for medical providers employed by chiropractors. I've been in many these offices and I've seen some that kept the appropriate line of authority in place, which is great and perfectly legitimate, and I've also seen offices where the chiropractor operated like a medical doctor, wore a white coat and presented themselves like a medical physician and discussed medical treatments with the patient, and of course selling expensive stem cell treatments.

Now take that environment of selling patients high-dollar stem cell treatments that aren't really stem cell treatments and you have a recipe for consumer fraud. This is what ultimately created the problems we saw in the stem cell treatment market several years ago, leading to wide scale industry restrictions. About ten years ago as of this writing, one company in particular coached hundreds of chiropractic offices on selling high dollar stem cell treatments. They advertised heavily and made a lot of promises. One of the popular phrases was "one-and-done" indicating that you only need one injection and the stem cells would heal your tissues and that's all you would ever need. It doesn't work that way with these products. The underlying condition the patient has is still there. These injections help but don't cure anything.

This was a huge problem that ultimately led the FDA and the FTC to crack down on unscrupulous offices making all sorts of claims and charging obscene amounts of money to "cure" medical problems using products that aren't actually stem cells.

I'm all about innovation and creativity, and if all this somehow actually helped advance stem cell medicine, I wouldn't complain, but it didn't advance the field, it damaged the reputation of the field and even drove Google and Facebook to ban ads for stem cell therapies under pressure from government regulators, yes, even for genuine stem cell therapies in legitimate offices, so it hurt everyone and set the whole industry back.

OK, I know I'm probably going a little too deep on this topic, but it's very important to understand this in terms of the condition of the stem cell market in the US because there's a reason you can only get certain types of stem cell therapy here in the US versus what's available around the world. BUT we are moving on in the world of stem cells to bigger and better things.

I just want those reading this to understand that history, because I still get this question from people all the time: what's the deal with chiropractors and stem cells? Now you know a little about that.

We are well on our way to standardizing the regenerative medicine world by collecting all this excellent data on concentration and outcomes. For instance, most of the doctors who offer you a PRP injection in their office are only going to be able to concentrate it in a range of three to four times the concentration it naturally occurs in the blood.

Will's Industry Insight #8:
Dose and concentration are everything! A quick note here on dosing, aka cell concentration. Standardization is the key ingredient in the future success of stem cell treatment.

Some companies have been compiling excellent documentation on the standardization of genuine stem cell and PRP therapies in the world. And guess what the secret ingredient is for healing success? Dosing!

You have to concentrate the treatment high enough to produce enough stimulation to induce the in-situ cells and tissues to heal. If you don't concentrate the dose, you won't get the outcomes, and there are studies showing just how much concentration is needed to obtain those outcomes.

What is the concentration needed to start seeing a huge difference in healing effect? Speaking to many providers and reviewing articles, 7x the normal concentration is the critical dose level to initiate efficacy, and 7x to 30x to get certain outcomes for certain tissues. This is all still in development and discovery with advances occurring all the time.

So, MOST doctors offering PRP are not even offering something that works on a significant therapeutic range. So, never make your choice based on price! The office down the street is going to claim to offer PRP cheaper, but they most likely aren't even in the same ballgame. Same for stem cells: you have to concentrate the dose to get the outcome.

That's why I love cultured expanded stem cell therapy, as I mentioned earlier. We can standardize this treatment and grow enough cells to concentrate the dose to create highly effective and successful outcomes. Dose and concentration are everything!

Amniotic membrane stem cells: The amniotic membrane is the actual sac that holds the fetus and fluid. It was one of the first tissues popularized for birth tissue stem cell use. The membrane is ideal because it has one of the lowest levels of immune markers on cell surfaces, nearly undetectable according to some research articles, so the risk of immune responses on recipients would be minimal to negligible.

Amniotic membrane patches: This happens to be an amazing wound care dressing for open wounds. It heals wounds and ulcers that are non-healing or difficult to treat. It's so good and so widely used that it's starting to become a standard of wound care treatment.

Most of these membranes are stripped of their cell content and dehydrated so it's not considered a stem cell product, but I've still heard it described to patients as a stem cell graft or a stem cell patch. It's not. It's just a dried piece of amniotic membrane with a lot of proteins that help tissues grow after being rehydrated on the wound. Still a great product for wound care though!

The amniotic membrane was used for numerous applications as a surgical dressing for burns and as an adjunctive tissue in surgical reconstruction of the oral cavity, bladder, and also for tympanoplasty, arthroplasty, repair of omphaloceles, and prevention of adhesions in pelvic and abdominal surgery.

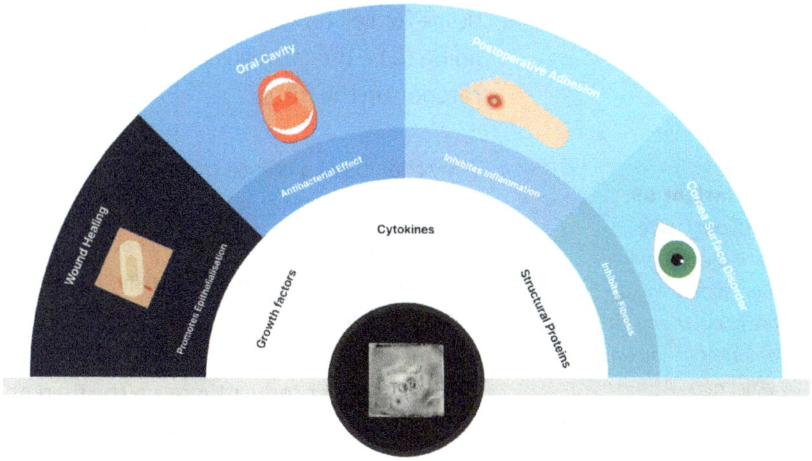

Amniotic Membrane Components, Characteristics, and Applications

An illustration of the amniotic membrane being vital for medical applications like burn dressings, tissue reconstruction, and preventing surgical adhesions.
Data from: https://www.mdpi.com/2077-0375/11/12/941

Cord blood stem cells: So, if I say blood, you say … hematopoietic. Correct! So, would these cells likely be used in your musculoskeletal treatment? There's a mix of cell types in cord blood, but ultimately cord blood stem cells for general regenerative medicine use and MSK use was heavily scrutinized a few years ago by the FDA and most of those operations were shut down quickly.

Labs were trying to find "the next best thing" to make and sell, but blood products are more complicated because they require blood type matching to be used, or they require more processing work to make them useful, so ultimately you only see cord blood stem cells in high-end medical research therapies like treating various cancers and organ damage. It's a very exciting category of stem cells, but not the pathway of musculoskeletal that I'm talking about here.

Cord tissue stem cells: This is the umbilical cord itself and all the tissue that makes it up. There's a good bit of cell content in this tissue that can be collected and used. Lately, it's been used as a great tissue source for doing mesenchymal stem cell culture and expansion work in international treatment programs, as the FDA in the US has clamped down on the injectable cord tissue product category.

Collecting the genuine mesenchymal cells out of this tissue for cell replication and expansion is probably going to be the most valuable aspect of this tissue category in the future.

Will's Industry Insight #9:
Cord tissue stem cells were popularized by a few companies looking to make something different from the more popular amniotic membrane products at the time, eight to 10 years ago.

What I know for certain, because I indirectly caused some of this required innovation, was that various researchers had non-compete contracts that prohibited them from working with amniotic membrane for any new company they worked for, so when those scientists left and worked for another company, or started their own labs, they couldn't work with amniotic membrane and instead worked with cord tissue.

They then had to create the industry perception that cord tissue was "better" or "newer" or "more advanced" than amniotic membrane, when there was no evidence of any superior quality other than that they could actually work with that tissue type under contract. (Just a little insight into why there are so many different product types on the market.) Yes, I've been involved in conversations with a lot of these labs and companies when they were starting and I've been offered a lot of positions and partnerships and all sorts of things to come over and help these new ventures get off the ground. So I know some of these very intimate industry insights.

Wharton's Jelly stem cells: Wharton's Jelly is the gelatinous cushion that surrounds the vessels in the umbilical cord. It's rich in cell content and is a great tissue category to work with.

Often people use the terms cord tissue and Wharton's Jelly interchangeably, and although there are differences between them, they are both still great tissues for this industry. Again, we still can't do injection products in the US like this anymore, but for a while it was very popular. It's also commonly used in research and for cell culture and expansion.

Placental stem cells: The placenta is another source of cells, but for reasons of complexity I won't go into more detail, but it's still a tissue type you see used in some capacity.

Whew! That's a lot of info for a short run through. I could literally talk about each one of these categories all day. I used to do this all the time: spend endless hours researching and reading all about the cellular biology of all these tissues and spend hours on the phone explaining these details to doctors, labs, other biotech start up groups, and investors of all kinds.

I've even been on the phone with the CEOs and medical directors of some of the top four major commercial health insurance companies discussing the possibilities of adding these product types to their covered treatments. They loved the idea, but the market needed to be more established for them.

Maybe in the future, but we're not there yet on reimbursement for these products. They were very interested though, and I had multiple calls with these groups and spent hours going over the fine details of these different products and the minutiae of differences between them.

I ultimately played the part of an expert witness to their legal departments over the risk of adding these products to their covered services, because ultimately it was their legal department that vetoed the use of these products as a covered benefit. They loved hearing about the outcomes and cost efficiency of reducing surgeries and invasive procedures by using these products. I'm sure I'll talk to them again one day when the market is ready for it.

Will's Industry Insight #10:
Minutiae of differences! Yep, as you can tell from the explanation above, there are a lot of minute details and differences between all these products. To make it even more complex, the FDA had categories to put all these products into and even those categories were nearly impossible for companies to interpret and distinguish.

Even today I hear of companies trying to make the case that their product is compliant in one category or another when, at the time of writing, the FDA has basically said none of these perinatal tissue products can be sold without now going through a drug trial, except amniotic membrane for wound covering. That's actually still a go and is reimbursable by Medicare and such, but everything else is non-compliant.

Even the companies making these products couldn't explain why their product wasn't the same as another or given the same status. I had one company's executive team attempt to debate me on how their product was compliant and I said to them, "I don't need to argue with you, I just need to see your FDA product compliance document – the paper that says your product is compliant under the category you're arguing about." They couldn't do it and they were really angry that I knew how to pin them down on this. In most of their sales conversations they can simply obfuscate the details enough to where the doctor just stops asking questions and believes them.

I don't mince words with these groups anymore because they still damage and discredit the market. I tell them that just because they make a product following the guidelines of that category does not mean it's compliant in that category, and claiming to be compliant and collecting money from sales based on that claim is fraud. That usually causes them all to pause for a few moments. I'm aiming for a real future in stem cell therapy so I can't suffer the fools who make us all look bad.

Will's Industry Insight #11:
Stem cells are a dirty word! Because of all the charlatans out there! The regulations have now shifted to what you can't say, based on the abuse of all the common terms or words used to describe.

Remember that what a doctor or chiropractor's office claims is stem cells that they pull out of the freezer is not stem cells nor is it necessarily what they say it is. It's most likely homogenized tissue injection that may contain a few viable stem cells at best, but it would be misleading to call it a stem cell injection, so regulations had to be enacted.

Stem cells are a pretty easy term to regulate, so the FDA basically said anyone claiming to offer stem cell treatments or injections is in violation, so they simply track down all the ads and websites claiming stem cells. Doctors and chiropractors would often change to another term to sell the same thing, so each new sales tactic resulted in another restricted word in the market. I've seen the progression of prohibited words keep going and going. The latest advertisement I saw for a company selling products to doctors offices called their product a beneficial injection. Using that term because no other word was allowed. So the advertisement encouraged doctors to call and learn more about what this beneficial injection does for your patient. Our beneficial injection is the best beneficial injection on the market. You can see how bad it's gotten when these companies can't use stem cells or any other birth tissue name, can't use regenerative medicine, can't say anything that indicates it's a biologic, and are reduced to just calling it a beneficial injection. It's pretty comical in some respects, but speaks to how all the bad actors out there have ruined the market. Stem cells are a dirty word now, but my goal is to bring a real and regulated stem cell therapy to the US medical field.

Chapter 2 – Non Stem Cell Products

(Primarily used in the US market)

So, what about non stem cell products and treatments? There are a lot of them, and I'll run through them quickly. They are not the same thing as any of these above stem cell type therapies, but they do work and most likely some of these therapies will be the first to market as FDA approved therapies that get covered by Medicare and commercial insurances.

Acellular amniotic fluid – pure fluid: Pure acellular amniotic fluid is amazing as a non stem cell product. Its outcomes are excellent and it's a very simple product to make and standardize. There are no cells to worry about, so you don't have to count cells or worry about viability, which means you don't have to validate or prove cell counts and viability in the lab process.

And remember what I said before: most doctors say their outcomes are roughly as good or even better with pure fluid versus a cellular based product. Remember all the reasons I mentioned before that a cellular product isn't what you think it is. Pure amniotic fluid is rich in growth factors and nutrients, and other beneficial things.

"Amniotic fluid is the perfect regenerative fluid mixture and the perfect regenerative medicine treatment because it's the biologically ideal mixture of components to support tissue growth and regeneration." – Will Bozeman.

Yep, I just quoted myself, but it's a true statement and I've been saying that for a decade now. The balance of growth factors and proteins is literally arranged in perfect ratios, so ultimately it would be the perfect fluid to use, no lab alteration required.

In fact, my most popular and successful product ever produced was the simplest version: pure amniotic fluid. We didn't alter it in any way; we simply filtered it for safety and left the concentrations exactly as is. This was the most successful regenerative product I've ever created in one of my biotech companies.

PRP (PRFM, A2M, platelet lysate, and other PRP isolates): Immediately I want to say that PRP is not all the same and what your doctor calls PRP in their office may be vastly different from PRP in another office under different processing techniques. Dosing and concentration are everything when it comes to PRP. Keep that in mind as I explain the basics here.

Platelet rich plasma was all the rage a couple of decades ago when a few high-end athletes mentioned getting PRP treatments for rapid recovery, which sparked a huge demand for PRP in the MSK field.

Then a few celebrities and influencers promoted PRP for facials and hair regeneration and then suddenly it was all the rage in esthetics – and still is. PRP is created by drawing your blood, spinning it down and concentrating the plasma, drawing that back out, and then reinjecting it into the damaged tissue. So, with all the processing techniques and processes out there, we can isolate almost any particular element out of your plasma and reinject that particular element instead of the whole plasma concoction.

This is an excellent advancement in regenerative medicine because all the studies show that different isolates of PRP are great at doing different things. So yeah, it can get complicated, and I won't go too far into the weeds on this, but I'll briefly mention the ones listed in the heading of this section.

PRP is platelet rich plasma and is simply concentrated plasma. PRFM is platelet rich fibrin matrix, which is simply PRP with a slightly different processing technique to make the mixture react differently and maybe more useful in some scenarios.

A2M is alpha-2-macroglobulin and is great at inhibiting cartilage deterioration by binding up the reactive proteins in your joints that cause cartilage deterioration.

Platelet lysate is one of the many isolates of PRP that can create enhanced healing effects on specific tissues. Again, the dosing is everything with each of these versions of PRP. Yeah, it gets complicated and there is a lot of research going into these various treatments. It's actively being proven that the concentrations of these treatments are just as important as what's in it.

In some studies a four times concentration of PRP does nearly nothing, while a seven times concentration crossed the threshold into tissue activity, all with the same stuff, just more concentrated. So don't worry too much about the particulars at the moment but know that when a doctor says "PRP," you want to know what exactly it is they are talking about. I'll give you some great pointers and questions to ask later.

Exosomes or secretomes: Exosomes are essentially the growth fluid used to grow stem cells in the lab. I create a plate of stem cells to grow in a dish and the nutrient rich fluid the cells need is used by the cells and the leftover fluid has a lot of the beneficial elements of the stem cell growth process.

After the cells start growing, they produce little micro lipid packets of signaling proteins that are excreted from the cell, called exosomes – because they exit the cell – and they're little enclosed lipid bodies like bubbles, so "exit-body" or the more scientifically sounding "exosome" fits the description. They're also called secretomes because they're secreted from the cell.

If stem cells are an apple orchard, exosomes are the truck loads of apples leaving the orchard.

The first lab to bring exosomes to market years ago was an associate of mine and we chatted a few times about the possibility of using this product. My first thought was that it could be a really interesting category, but it wasn't even a market category at all, so how would it be viewed by regulators and the medical community? I didn't know at all. I told them it sounded interesting, but it would be an unknown risk to bring it to market.

Fast-forward a couple years and they were selling across the nation, and a dozen other groups were making their own exosome products. So, exosomes were all the hype for a few years and got a lot of negative attention, and, ultimately, you don't see them much anymore.

Exosomes are still around, but they got hammered by the FDA for misrepresentation because sales reps and companies were selling them under the wrong terms. They started out calling them stem cells like everything else, but when stem cells became a dirty word, they switched to calling exosomes amniotic fluid. Why? Let me throw in a little Will's Industry Insight here to explain.

Keep in mind, I was on the phone with the top executives at this biotech company: the CEO, their Chief Medical Officer, their Chief Science Officer, and their Chief Sales Officer. They were the ones who were deciding how to educate their clients, doctors, on what this product was that they were selling.

I said, "What you're describing is not amniotic fluid, it's exosomes."

Long pause. "Yeah, we know it's actually exosomes but," here are their own words and I wish I had recorded this, "it's too difficult to educate doctors on the nuances of different products, so we just call it amniotic fluid because they understand that and it's more acceptable to them."

So, there you have it: the reason for all the regulations and problems we've had in the regenerative medicine industry over the last five years. You can't call it what it isn't. So, after they got caught calling it the wrong thing, which I thoroughly warned them about, they were forced to change their description type to a new term, "amniotic derived fluid," which again, was all to avoid calling it what it actually was: exosomes.

All this was because it was too hard to explain exosomes and there were already major competitors in the market for exosomes and they wanted something unique that couldn't be replicated by competitors. So, this company thought they'd be clever and create a new market category, but the FDA moved all lab grown products into another classification later and that basically stopped everyone in their tracks on exosomes.

Will's Industry Insight #12:
A company reached out to me a year after exosomes were in the market wanting my help on distribution and growth with their new "unique amniotic fluid" product line.

I asked them a few questions because amniotic fluid was an official unique product designation, meaning it's not like anything else and the FDA recognizes this as a unique thing, which means you can't change it without calling it something else … meaning your brand of amniotic fluid can't be "unique amniotic fluid" and still be compliant.

They told me they were growing amniotic fluid in the lab. I asked how they were doing that because amniotic fluid doesn't grow in labs. They said they were culturing stem cells and taking the growth fluid and making amniotic fluid because they were using amniotic membrane stem cells and that's what amniotic fluid was, right? Simple logic … right? The fluid spins off from the amniotic membrane? You can see how complicated the definitions can be.

Peptides: This is an exciting new field of medicine with a lot of potential. Peptides are protein compound segments that are created to affect certain cellular responses. Stem cells are the orchard, exosomes are the apples, and peptides are the juice in the apples. Cells are looking for the signals from other cells to communicate and take actions.

Peptides are great because they can be grown in the lab and all sorts of specific peptides can be isolated and grown in concentration. I believe there is exceptional biologic standardization potential with peptides, so I'm actively keeping an eye on peptides and looking forward to the innovation in that field.

Prolotherapy: Prolotherapy is a dextrose sugar injection that agitates the tissues at the cellular level and creates a mild inflammation with a healing effect afterwards, like doing an exfoliating scrub on your face to remove all the dead skin and the after effect creates fine, smooth skin.

Some physicians wouldn't call prolotherapy a true regenerative medicine therapy in the same category as these other items above, but many do feel that it qualifies as a regenerative.

It's great of course, but you're not adding any regenerative elements to this process, you're simply agitating tissue to become mildly inflamed and then letting it heal back up. In short, it's simply creating a mild local tissue irritation through dextrose sugar crystals roughing up the cells and tissue and causing inflammation and mild tissue damage in that area for the cells to be agitated and triggered into healing.

I've talked to doctors who do consider it regenerative, but I've talked to a lot of doctors about this and with all the better options out there, stem cells, PRP, and other options, it's hard to justify doing old school prolotherapy except that it's so affordable because dextrose is really cheap, and the injections are very simple and easy.

That's the wrap up on the general overview of regenerative medicine in the US. Keep in mind that by the time you read this, some of the things I mentioned may have new regulations and you may not find some of these options at all.

Now, let's talk about osteoarthritis and how regenerative medicine treatments are changing the entire treatment strategy for this condition. You have options, and stem cells for osteoarthritis may be exactly what you need!

Chapter 3 – All About Osteoarthritis

Osteoarthritis (OA) has existed from the beginning of time, diagnosed in the shoulders and spines of Egyptian mummies. However, it wasn't until Sir Edward Archibald Garrod in 1890 that osteoarthritis was defined and made distinct from other forms of arthritis.

Osteoarthritis is described as a wear-and-tear condition. It's a deterioration of a joint from just using it over and over for years and years. This is why it stays persistently common in the population, despite all the efforts to treat it.

Rheumatoid arthritis (RA) is an autoimmune condition where the joint is attacked and damaged through inflammatory processes. Most people are familiar with hearing about both of these types; however, as OA is a result of joint tissues wearing down over time, it becomes a prime treatment target for regenerative medicine!

In 2018 Dr. Christopher Centeno, MD, and his associates concluded that, "[i]n the United States, symptomatic OA affects more than 50 million adults, resulting in annual costs due to medical expenses and lost wages exceeding $100 billion." Yes, that's the annual cost of osteoarthritis in the US alone!

However, due to multiple compounding risk factors and an increasingly aged population, cases of OA have increased significantly over the past few years. So, we should expect to see those figures increase over the coming decades.

What should be understood by readers is that the size of the baby boomer population has contributed significantly to the increase in OA cases. Because of this, OA has been recognized as the fastest increasing health condition and disability in the world.

More than 10% of the world's population has experienced or will experience the effects of OA, including its various side effects that can change the way they respond to daily tasks. Although the percentage of the population over 60 years old with osteoarthritis has remained static, the increase in the aged population contributes to a larger total number of OA cases.

According to the CDC and physicians like Kamil Barbour, by the year 2040, 78 million patients will be diagnosed with some form of arthritis. More than ever, OA presents a unique challenge, not only for the aging population but for all who search for an effective treatment. (Osteoarthritis Action Alliance)

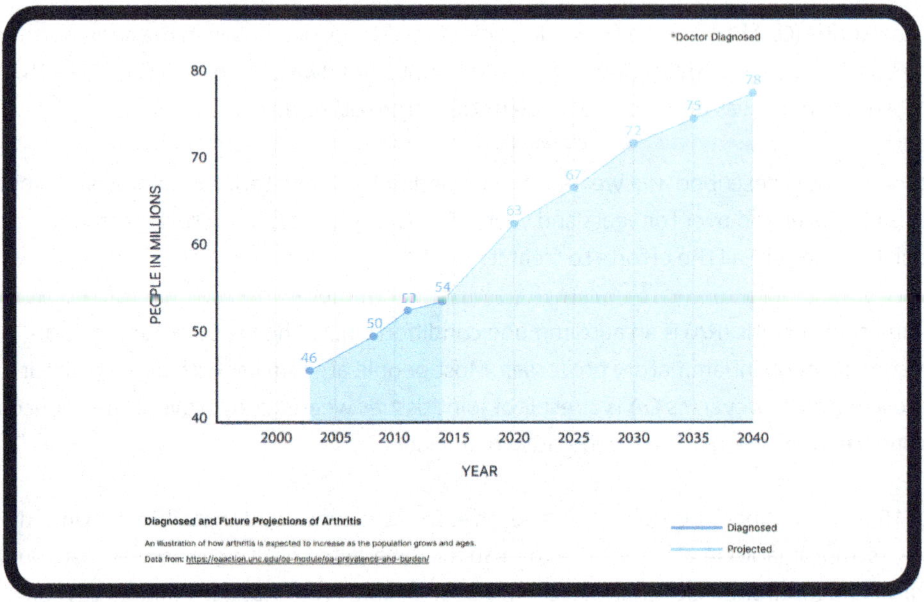

Because of the increase in OA cases and their severity, decades of research and millions of dollars have been spent in the pursuit of an effective and safe treatment. Osteoarthritis is also a pain condition, so people will only suffer through it for so long before they take action.

The question now is what actions are viable for patients and likely to work to relieve pain, and then attempt to resolve the symptoms. There aren't very many good options available for this condition. Also, keep in mind that because it is a wear and tear condition, it's not going to go away, even with all the treatment efforts.

Ultimately, the risk involved with conventional treatments, ranging from over the counter painkillers to surgery, doesn't leave patients with many long-term viable options. And like most patients know, the path of knee osteoarthritis is also the path to knee replacement surgery, and that path doesn't always lead to success and relief. In fact, there are studies that show the success rate of knee replacements is quite low compared to how highly they are promoted as a treatment option for knee OA. Alternatively, you can do a few temporary treatments to stave off the inevitable knee replacement, but there's not much available.

Also, other joints with OA may have even fewer options. More and more evidence supports the use of stem cells to treat OA but before patients can understand how stem cells treat OA, I'll finish going over a few details about the condition.

Osteoarthritis is considered a wear-and-tear condition, meaning that it's a factor of the joint and cartilage just getting worn down over time and the internal anatomy of the joint is damaged due to continued wearing down. Most of the time, osteoarthritis presents with symptoms of bone spurs, stiffness, and pain. It's also common to see cases where patients suffer from osteoarthritis in conjunction with other debilitating conditions.

So, OA may simply be one of several problems a patient is dealing with. What this means is that medications and surgeries that are meant to treat the OA condition may make other conditions worse. However, as I mentioned before, OA is also a pain condition, so people don't usually wait too long to get help. Also, movement is a key ingredient in health and longevity, so if you can't move easily or can't move because of pain, then you're more sedentary and everything will keep getting worse. This is another reason people seek out treatment.

Treating osteoarthritis is a critical step to getting patients' overall health back on track. It's common for one problem to intermingle with another, as is the case with OA; if you can treat it effectively, you can improve a lot of other things indirectly.

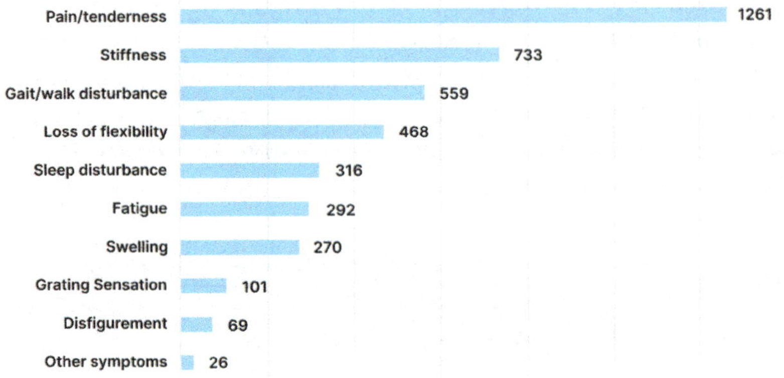

Common Osteoarthritis Symptoms Reported by Patients

This graph provides an overview of the key symptoms of osteoarthritis symptoms as well as their prevalence

Data from: https://bmcmusculoskeletdisord.biomedcentral.com/articles/10.1186/s12891-020-03741-0

The earliest signs of osteoarthritis are not as difficult to deal with, so it takes time for patients to seek out treatment. It's more likely that patients will experience a chain reaction of symptoms that play off one another: stiffness leading to strained flexibility, which leads to pain, swelling, and worsened stiffness.

It's no surprise that patients with OA experience profound frustration, not only at the lack of effective treatment, but at this chain of reactive symptoms that trigger in response to any form of physical activity.

Now you're starting to see why the drive toward stem cells for osteoarthritis is so attractive. Stem cells may be the only genuine treatment for OA, seeing how it is a progressive disease with limited prevention.

Barring surgery, there is little physicians and patients can do to maintain the cartilage that is worn down in the joints. When the cartilage wears down, and it is literally only a matter of time before it does, osteoarthritis and all its symptoms are the result.

For a simple and clear picture of the wearing down process, it might be useful to picture the cartilage between our joints as brake pads that keep our bones from grinding together. The harder we are on our joints – the more we use our bodies' brake pads – the quicker we will develop osteoarthritis.

Besides age, there are other risk factors I will mention later that contribute to the pathogenesis of this condition. For now, it is useful that patients understand the condition itself, how to recognize it, and where it might show its existence.

Types and Locations of Osteoarthritis

While the unfortunate reality is that osteoarthritis can appear in most joints, depending on their use and associated risk factors, more often than not, a typical case of osteoarthritis that first appears in patients over the age of fifty is generally located in the knees, hands, and hips – as demonstrated in Professor David Hunter's chart below.

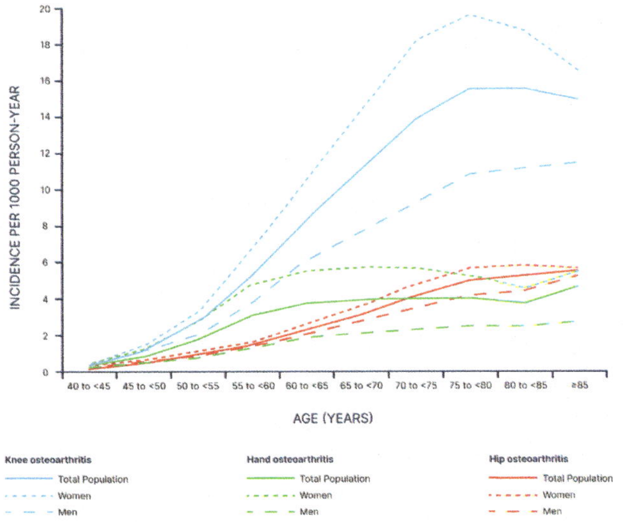

Prevalence Across Age Groups and Joint Types Over Time

An illustration of the population distribution of knee, hand, and hip osteoarthritis according to age and diagnosis on an annual basis.
Data from: https://www.thelancet.com/journals/lancet/article/PIIS0140-6736%2819%2930417-8/fulltext

We all understand the vital importance of joint movement and flexibility, and there is no denying we all maintain a heavy reliance on these joints to accomplish regular, everyday activities. Some, if not the ***most***, crucial joints that we use every day are hips, hands and knees.

Because of the natural anatomical reliance on our feet, anything that affects the ability of our feet will greatly affect our quality of life. Most people are familiar with referred pain and understand that a problem in your knee can trigger pain in your hip and foot. If the hip or knee joints experience pain, the consequences of this pain may extend to your feet and suddenly your quality of life in general is negatively affected.

As you can see from the graph on the following page, knees are the most commonly affected, which is why knees get the most attention in the conversation about osteoarthritis. (Hunter et al, 2019)

Despite the high prevalence of knee osteoarthritis, we likely have a lot more activity associated with our hands. Most patients suffering from hand osteoarthritis are familiar with its four phases, defined by their levels of pain – from mild to severe. Regardless of the phase a patient experiences, limited capability with the hands is always a factor in quality of life and the ability to do nearly everything.

On a similar level of occurrence as hand osteoarthritis, though more common with increased age, is hip osteoarthritis. This type of osteoarthritis, though less common than knee osteoarthritis, retains similar risk factors and pathogenesis. Virtually all risk factors associated with knee OA – including obesity, age, and injury – also apply to hip OA.

This association between hip and knee OA and not hand OA might help patients understand why preventative measures and treatment vary. For example, risk factors like obesity can be adjusted as a preventative measure against knee and hip osteoarthritis, but the same cannot be said for hand OA. Although these types of osteoarthritis vary, the impacts they have on a patient's mobility and quality of life are no less important.

When comparing the knee joint to the hip and hand joints, the knee is most vulnerable and at risk for OA pathogenesis. It is vulnerable to being hit, knocked, and twisted, while bearing the load of the human body, so it would follow that it is typically the joint most affected by osteoarthritis.

Because of the increased risk inherent with the knee, focus on this joint has only increased. Physicians and patients should try to correctly diagnose early signs of the condition so they can apply as many interventions as possible to prevent the severity. It's important that patients receive a medical diagnosis of their condition, and patients will need this official diagnosis to move forward on any therapies offered.

It might not be surprising for readers to know that many patients with knee osteoarthritis exhibit the condition as a direct result of sports and athletics in their younger years. Young patients participating in sports directly contribute to the increase in knee cartilage loss and early onset osteoarthritis. It's a wear and tear condition, so it takes a while to occur, but it starts with heavy usage in the younger years.

Without proper training, physical exercise, and injury avoidance measures, athletes (both young and old) are at greater risk for knee osteoarthritis, which in conventional terms means they are at greater risk of knee surgeries and knee replacements later in life. At the same time, consistent healthy, safe exercise can provide a lifetime of healthy knee joints.

Most experts agree that vigorous walking is great exercise and a good replacement for higher impact actions like running or sports with a lot of start and stop motions like basketball and tennis, where the knee is absorbing all the impact of the start and stop cycle over and over.

Healthy knee joints should allow for a highly flexible range of motion, permitting the movement of our legs, depending on knee joint health and practiced flexibility. The rotation and flexibility of our legs depend on a group of muscles and tendons that keeps our knees in their sockets.

As we increase in age and acquire more risk factors for osteoarthritis, the range of motion in our knees decreases drastically. However, knee joint health and its level of pain will also depend on the aforementioned condition of the muscles surrounding the joint – muscles that can be improved and maintained via physical exercise.

However, muscle inflammation can also contribute to the pain a patient experiences in their joints. In fact, the most common cause of knee pain can be tied back to the inflation of these muscles as they press against the bones of the knee.

In an equal yet distinct way, bone spurs (which occur largely in the elderly with osteoarthritis) can grow on the bones in the knee and press against these muscles. Other causes of knee pain include dislocation, overuse, and even bad posture. Not only will patients with OA experience a higher level of pain around their joints but they will also experience less flexibility due to stiffness in the joints as a result of inflammation.

One of the strongest signs of pain is inflammation but inflammation is a response to injury and the two can bounce back and forth in a negative feedback loop. Pain is essential for the body as it is the body's first response to a problem and triggers an effort to promote healing and recovery.

Most people can recognize the moment they stub their toe or nick a finger and the ensuing pain is underway. There's that awkward moment before you feel the pain when you know it's coming and you're just waiting for it. I have literally done this before: banged a toe and simply waited for the pain to hit, knowing it's about to happen.

Within a split second, pain manifests itself to tell us something must be done on our end to address the injury. Usually, it's to protect the injury; however, pain should also be seen as a signal that our system is doing its part to fix the problem. Inflammation is the same signal process, triggering a response from us to take action.

The problem with chronic pain conditions is that despite the pain and inflammation, your body is no longer metabolically agile enough to rapidly heal the damage you're being warned about. This is why chronic conditions like osteoarthritis need a treatment that replaces or amplifies the healing process because your body isn't going to be able to step up and handle it on its own. Again, now you can see how stem cell therapy can potentially change how we treat osteoarthritis and chronic pain conditions.

While signs of pain and inflammation occur around the joints as a trigger to rest while the body heals, stiffness and reduced flexibility are common onsets of lack of movement and often the need to sit still creates even more downward cycles, which is understandably frustrating. Consequently, if a patient is able to treat and prevent osteoarthritis pain, they will also prevent the associated inflammation and ultimately maintain flexibility.

When patients understand the cause and effect of pain and inflammation resulting from OA – side effects like reduced flexibility and increased pain and swelling – they can begin to understand that it may need a total joint reset to get it back into desirable operating conditions.

It sounds a lot like how experts for decades have determined that the ultimate fate of an OA knee is to have a knee replacement, or for a hip, a hip replacement. You can't just keep treating the symptoms with over the counter meds; you eventually have to overhaul the problem and start over. I think this is where stem cell therapy for osteoarthritis becomes the new, better, and best option.

My advice is that if you're going to go through the effort and expense of having a stem cell treatment for chronic OA, you should prepare for this therapy by adjusting your lifestyle to get the full and complete benefit out of the treatment.

Eat better, get more exercise that is healthy and safe, spend more quality time on positive activities with friends and family to improve your mental outlook, get better sleep, take proper supplements to bridge your nutritional deficiencies (healthy eating can be better than supplements and can bridge that nutrition gap), and stay well hydrated.

Will's Industry Insight #13:
Chronic conditions are called chronic for a reason, and they aren't going to be "cured" but simply managed as well as possible. Most of the time, the lifestyle choices being engaged in are triggering or exacerbating a chronic condition like OA, and even with a great option like stem cell therapy, the underlying chronic problem remains and will need to be addressed.

Also, consider getting tested for things that your doctor isn't going to help you with because your doctor may not think there's an immediate need for it, not a "medical necessity" for it, though it could still be beneficial. Get sleep tested, get allergy tested, get heavy metal tested, and consider getting tested for things you're not hearing much about like your gut microbiome.

There are a lot of things that can improve your overall health and make your big treatments and procedures more successful. Stem cell therapy for knee, hip, and hand osteoarthritis is the future of medicine, but you still have to take care of yourself and your underlying conditions in all areas, to make those treatments effective and last as long as possible.

Risk Factors, Intervention, and Conventional Treatment Options

The steady percentage and high volume of OA cases has contributed to a steady and persistent level of research into a treatment for this condition. (Anandacoomarasamy & March, 2010) Unfortunately, research from several in the medical community concludes that effective treatment for osteoarthritis is still unknown, elusive, and often lacks the desired outcomes by both patients and their doctors. Oddly enough, the newer generation of doctors will be the ones who take stem cell treatments seriously, while the older generation typically holds to the traditional therapies.

There's an excellent book on this concept I read before medical school that really influenced my thoughts on the advancement of science and medicine called ***The Structure of Scientific Revolutions***. This book outlines the process for new and innovative concepts to be adopted by the science and medical communities.

It's basically a process of rotating out the experts in the field and replacing them with new experts who are younger and whose opinions are not fixed on past concepts or resting their expertise on what you can't do rather than what you can do.

Keep in mind that it is absolutely essential for medicine to be a "big ship" that takes a long time to change course. This is how medicine stays safe and effective because we don't have thousands of doctors shooting from the hip on thousands of abstract ideas for healing and treating patients.

Standardization is the hallmark of modern medicine because this allows us to use actual data and scientific method to create standardized treatments, which is why it's good for doctors to question new therapies, beat up new and current ideas, and resist change to the point that a therapy has to prove itself to win these doctors over.

If not for this method, we'd be bombarded with chaotic therapy options and doctors who base their decisions on whims and emotional states. We can't structure modern medicine this way, so in order for new concepts like stem cell therapy to be implemented into mainstream medicine, it has to be standardized and formalized into data-driven structured therapies. This is exactly what I have been working on for the last decade in the biotech space. Now, I'm still working on it with stem cell therapy trials that are attempting to standardize treatment outcomes for a range of conditions.

I just wanted to point this out as I review the conventional therapies and explain why they are going to stick around for a while despite seemingly better options in stem cell therapy.

Unfortunately, as is the case for many conditions, there is no actual cure for osteoarthritis yet. There are only treatments for the condition that can help manage the pain and improve joint and limb functionality. Because developments in treating OA continue, and none are ideal solutions for the condition, many physicians and their patients propose placing an increased emphasis on preventative measures like I mentioned above.

However, many patients who are past the point of prevention will likely not accept that as an answer when they are in pain and actively fighting a daily battle with OA. However, this is exactly what I've mentioned before: if you're going to proceed with a stem cell treatment, then take care of that treatment with lifestyle changes that prevent continued OA degradation. So, once you have OA, you have to deal with it, and prevention is too late at that point.

While the concept of preventative measures has received less attention than the more drastic measures like knee and hip replacements, there can be no doubt that their association with risk factors and their mitigation is paramount in the maintenance of a patient's quality of life.

While patients assess their risk factors, including age and obesity, they may be able to determine their likelihood of worsening their already diagnosed condition. Again, there's a point where you have to decide what you're going to do: make changes, get a major treatment – or, ideally, both.

When conducting a 2016 study, Dr. Carlen Reyes and her associates determined the likelihood of knee osteoarthritis, dependent on patients' age and weight. Doctors can see with clarity that the increase in incidence is directly correlated with patients' level of obesity and their age.

This study suggests that subsequent to patients reaching 40 years of age, there is an increase in the exhibited symptoms and diagnosis of osteoarthritis. After 40, patients with osteoarthritis only have worsening symptoms with OA as they climb into their 70s and 80s.

However, it is clear that not only does age have an impact on the incidence of osteoarthritis but obesity has a sharp influence on OA incidence. After all, more weight on the joint presses harder on the cartilage, making the wear and tear occur faster. Not only did these doctors determine that obesity directly and considerably affects knee osteoarthritis but hip, and even hand OA as well.

In the end it was determined that if patients and their doctors would like to see a decrease in the severity of osteoarthritis, the preventative measures of weight loss and exercise should be implemented early and often. It's never too late to work on being healthier.

Now, imagine that a stem cell treatment gave you that chance to reverse the clock on your joint and you were able to start making those necessary preventative changes. This is what stem cell therapy can offer: a chance to recapture those preventative efforts.

Patients may protest that age is a risk factor that cannot be overcome. I'll address this issue in other books dealing with the concept of longevity and aging; however, there are risk factors that can be addressed to mitigate the worsening of OA.

As mentioned previously, the risk factor of weight is highly adjustable and capable of reduction. Knowing that this particular risk factor contributes highly to the pathogenesis of osteoarthritis but that it can be actively reduced gives hope to patients. The best way to avoid worsening effects of OA is to reduce the manageable and changeable risk factors as soon as possible.

It's also possible that patients who attempt to reduce their body weight through exercise might trigger other risk factors that could worsen the OA pain. Afterall, use of the joint has caused OA, so exercising would impact the symptoms.

I mention often that patients need safe and healthy exercise that doesn't impact the joints too much. Exercising in an attempt to reduce weight can be an important method for OA management. While a patient reduces their weight through diet and exercise, muscles are built to maintain and protect joint functionality.

Elderly patients hearing this advice should not take offense or feel discouraged against exercise, as it is the same advice that would be given to young athletes who also bear the risk of developing OA from sports-related injuries.

All patients should exercise to decrease their current comorbidities, such as obesity, and understanding how to exercise properly could be the difference. I'm not going to outline all the exercise options here, but a good trainer at your local gym, or a recommendation from a physical therapist can probably help you get on a good, safe exercise program. Just off the top of my head, some lower impact exercises are water aerobics and cycling.

Conventional Treatments for Osteoarthritis

We definitely need effective nonsurgical treatment options for osteoarthritis. Even professionals in the medical community are frustrated at the lack of effective, safe and simple options available to their patients. Many available options, with their limited benefits and numerous side-effects, will make anyone conclude that there is a dire need for more safe and effective treatments for osteoarthritis.

Throughout the survey of treatments, physicians everywhere conclude that some drugs had little to no effect in a clinical trial when compared to the effects of a placebo. It's perhaps most disappointing to hear that even as our understanding of osteoarthritis and its painful side effects increases, we have very little to show when it comes to an effective treatment, until we consider stem cell therapy, which I will outline below after I walk through a review of a few of the most common therapies being offered.

Nutraceuticals
One of the most common and simple nonsurgical treatments for OA are special supplements and nutraceuticals. Nutraceuticals are supplements that claim to have an impact on a certain condition like OA, for example.

Nutraceuticals should improve the life and health of an individual when being taken for a certain condition and when used in tandem with healthy foods. The general assumption is that nutraceutical efficacy works in tandem with the patient's willingness to live a healthy lifestyle.

The most common nutraceuticals offered for OA include glucosamine sulfate, chondroitin methylsulfonylmethane (often combined as glucosamine chondroitin with MSM), fish oils like cod liver oil and derivatives of oils, and many others. There are many more that I won't go into because this book prioritizes modern stem cell therapy, not supplements.

The efficacy of nutraceutical treatments has been debated among peers in the medical community for decades. Notwithstanding, many physicians have limited non-invasive options, so they are prone to agree to most simple therapies that are considered generally safe for use, and they often recommend a range of supplements because there's usually no harm in trying these and crossing your fingers for useful outcomes.

The fact is that regulations surrounding nutraceuticals, their safety, and their efficacy are still under review. This is in part due to the medical community's skepticism of nutraceuticals claims from unscrupulous companies trying to compete in the market.

Not to throw too much shade on this category, but I'm sure you've seen every trick in the book to get you to buy a supplement, from wild claims to celebrity endorsements and multi-level marketing schemes. The product doesn't even have to work to get some people excited about it because they are not excited about the product but making money selling it. So, that whole multi-level marketing category of nutraceuticals can be dismissed as wrongly incentivized, skewed data because you can't believe anything being published where the intent is selling people on selling.

The FDA pays attention to claims as a way to regulate this industry, so companies have to be really careful about making claims of effectiveness or practically any claim related to a condition or an outcome. However, nutraceuticals are still being considered by governmental bodies as they continue to educate the public and the medical community on the benefits.

Understandably, skepticism continues to be a persistent issue and it will require in-depth clinical studies to validate the claims these companies make about their products.

With the efficacy, safety, and the various claims of all the many nutraceuticals available, it will require more evidence to make these a standard treatment modality. Many will likely find that nutraceuticals such as glucosamine have little to no effect on OA pain. The consensus of the people I have talked to is that nutraceuticals are more in line with preventative measures rather than treating a live and active condition, especially when a patient is in daily pain.

These conclusions on the benefits of nutraceuticals are a little disappointing and frustrating, especially for those who need a non-surgical and non-opioid treatment. This does help me make the case for what I believe is the future standard of care for OA: stem cell joint injections using either bone marrow collected stem cells or cultured expanded cells.

Physiotherapy

Also known as physical therapy, physiotherapy can be a relatively effective method for treating osteoarthritis. Because of physiotherapy's multifaceted and multistage-focused approach, patients can maintain flexibility and reduce pain from their osteoarthritis.

Physiotherapy focuses not only on treatment of pain but preventative measures and rehabilitation as well. For physiotherapy specifically, the method for treatment through these stages of OA includes extensive exercise and the use of biomechanical support, such as compression devices and braces.

For all intents and purposes, physiotherapy presents evidence that it is moderately effective in treating OA symptoms; however, there is also evidence to suggest it may be more supplementary than curative. Remember that it's a chronic condition and physiotherapy is only going to manage some of the symptoms for a short time before it continues to degrade.

While physical therapy exercises have a strong track record of short-term effects like decreased pain and increased function, there is little patients can do to maintain these effects in the long term. Other than implementing these exercises in a daily routine, which on its own can be difficult to maintain, it is likely that patients will need to supplement their physiotherapy with other treatment methods to treat osteoarthritis pain. However, delivery methods used to implement this therapy are increasing and improving.

Patients don't need to rely solely on individual exercise; they have options for home visits and group work to help motivate them and maintain consistency. I've talked to several doctors about the benefits of group work, and they report that group activities really motivate patients. Because adherence to this treatment via a strict regimen is essential for maintaining a quality of life and managing pain, various delivery methods to suit patients' needs are essential.

Essentially, physiotherapy and its efficacy in treating osteoarthritis is directly linked to a patient's adherence and dedication to the prescribed exercises. If patients are unwilling or unable to maintain consistent exercise, it is likely that they will see a decrease in the efficacy of physiotherapy. Again, this is a temporary therapy, so patients will need something else eventually.

In reality, a patient who maintains consistent exercise and uses biomechanical technology to help support their OA-affected joints will see the best results and manage the most pain. Evidence is clear that physiotherapy can be an effective and manageable temporary treatment for osteoarthritis. In reality, I see this as being a placeholder for other future therapies. Physiotherapy isn't going to regenerate the damaged tissue, so you'll still need something more substantial down the road, which again, is where I see expanded stem cell therapy as the future standard of care for OA.

Icing

Any patient familiar with muscle soreness knows that icing the affected area will result in a temporary decrease in inflammation and this is often the same when the pain is a result of OA inflammation. You can easily see that this isn't really a solution, but if you don't have much else, this is at least something.

Over the counter meds and NSAIDs

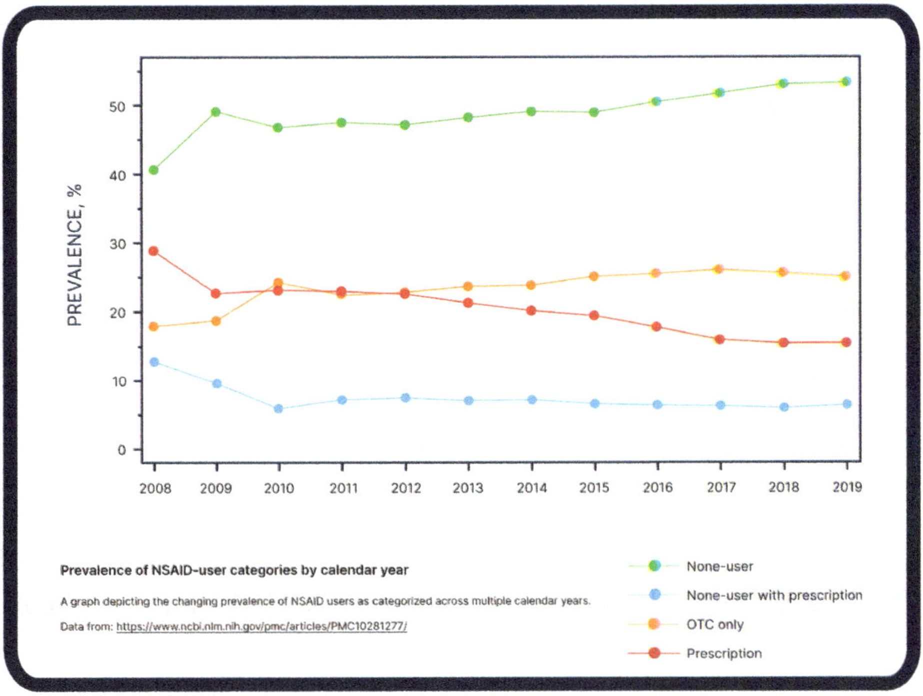

Prevalence of NSAID-user categories by calendar year

A graph depicting the changing prevalence of NSAID users as categorized across multiple calendar years.

Data from: https://www.ncbi.nlm.nih.gov/pmc/articles/PMC10281277/

Acetaminophen, aspirin, naproxen, ibuprofen and more are all over the counter household drugs with a range of symptom relief and capabilities, all of which are short-term and temporarily effective therapies. Some of these fall into the category of NSAIDs, non-steroidal anti-inflammatory drugs. (Magni et al 2021)

For early treatment of osteoarthritis pain, these medications can work decently well for a few hours at a time. The problem is that people tend to take them too often and at too high a dose for safe long-term use and they become "dependent," so this can create its own set of problems. I say dependent with inverted commas because it's not so much a problem of becoming addicted as much as a problem of making these drugs your go-to treatment and using them too much. Also, over the counter meds tend to lose their efficacy over time and require higher doses to maintain the effect. Studies evaluating the efficacy of these meds have also shown troubling side effects such as gastrointestinal and cardiovascular toxicity.

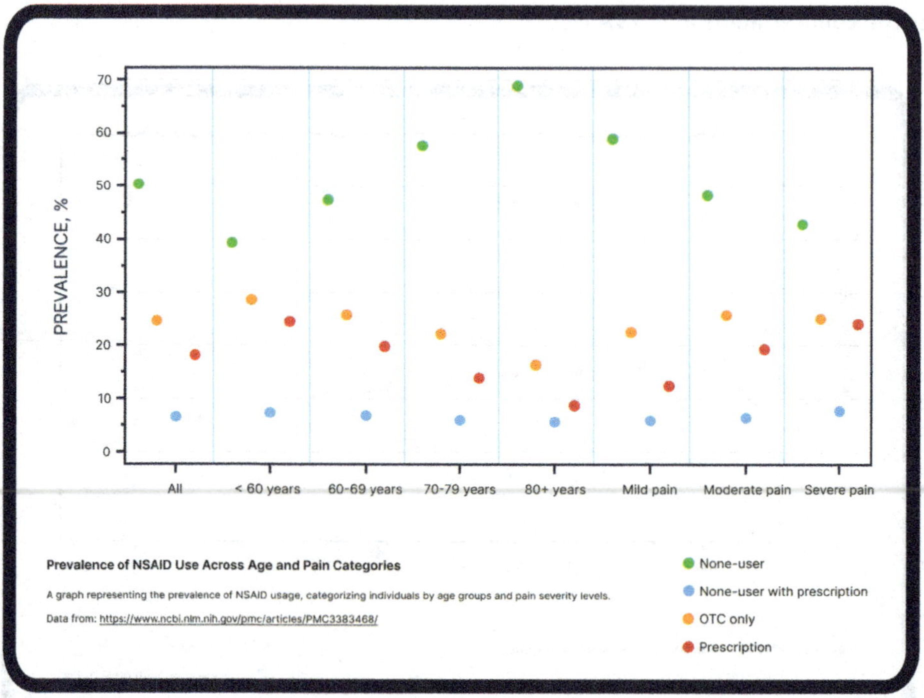

NSAIDs are known to cause gastrointestinal lining issues and ulcers and other pretty bad side effects, and acetaminophen is known to cause liver failure if a patient overdoses. For these reasons, it is important that all patients suffering from OA pain do not develop an over-dependence on over the counter painkillers and NSAIDs without considering the side-effects and complications they may cause. If patients are not careful, their overuse of these drugs can lead to more urgent problems that will be worse than the OA pain they're trying to treat.

In our studies, particularly in relation to the use of NSAIDs as a supplement to other forms of treatment, NSAIDs still have their place. I don't want to beat them up too much because they are a simple solution in a pinch. I will consider some of the pros related to NSAIDs as they are used jointly with other treatment options. NSAIDs are predominantly safe and therefore readily available to most of the population, and while these drugs can provide temporary relief, there are other effects that should be considered by patients.

While not directly addictive to patients who take NSAIDs to deal with OA pain, there's still a concern of ongoing use and overuse, so be aware of that. Dr. Centeno, in his 2018 study examining osteoarthritis treatments, concluded that NSAIDs, "[...] are not curative and [are] associated with side effects when used long term, including upper gastrointestinal complications and increased risk of cardiovascular events."

The effects of NSAIDs, while often effective at treating pain temporarily, are ephemeral and do not last long enough for patients to experience relief over a long period of time. Patients who experience OA pain for long periods of time will know that NSAIDs are not going to be a lasting treatment for their pain. However, when used in conjunction with other treatment methods, NSAIDs may provide relief long enough for patients to work through life situations and aim for additional, more substantial treatments.

The minor efficacy of NSAIDs can easily cause overuse and ongoing use. I personally know people who add an extra pill to their dose after a while, to ease the pain. Dependency and even overdose are real factors.

Just to clarify, overdose with NSAIDs is not like overdose with opioids that everyone is familiar with from the news. It doesn't result in death or comatose events, but more often overuse resulting in an adverse effect as mentioned above. With that in mind, the mild nature of NSAIDs often leads to heavier doses outside of the recommendation, which is a dangerous step that should not be considered when treating osteoarthritis pain.

One of these trade-offs of NSAIDs was critiqued in 2012 by the New Zealand Medicine and Medical Devices Safety Authority and categorized as, "[...] severe cutaneous adverse reactions (SCARs)." (New Zealand Government 2012) The researchers conclude that, "SCARs include bullous eruptions, erythema multiforme, epidermal necrolysis, toxic epidermal necrolysis and Stevens Johnson syndrome. The Centre for Adverse Reactions Monitoring (CARM) has received a number of reports of SCARs associated with NSAIDs."

Moreover, this research attests to the fact that these SCARs have been directly tied to NSAIDs and that SCARs, "[...] may cause permanent sequelae such as disfigurement, blindness and death. Importantly, these reactions may occur without warning." Although the research also suggests that the risk of NSAID-induced SCARs are low, these researchers were able to determine that, "In New Zealand, the NSAIDs most commonly reported to cause SCARs are piroxicam, naproxen, diclofenac, celecoxib and ibuprofen."

Although the risk of SCARs is low for patients who choose to use NSAIDs for routine pain treatment, there is a necessity to emphasize this risk for patient awareness. An over dependence on NSAIDs for treatment without consideration for alternatives could lead to dangerous consequences.

The pros and cons of NSAID treatment are great examples of the limited options available for OA pain. Patients around the world have learned to trust the quick relief offered by these drugs. This is why I keep coming back to what I believe is the future of medical treatment for OA: the new advancement of high dose stem cells.

As we move on and explore additional conventional treatment options for osteoarthritis, patients should consider them objectively, recognizing both the pros and cons of each. I also encourage you to think about how there is a better option that wasn't available even a decade ago, so my intent is to drive everyone in the medical field in the direction of stem cell therapy being the new standard of care for OA.

Radiologic grades of knee X-rays.

Grade	Grade of Degeneration
0:	normal joint
1:	osteophytes, osteosclerosis
2:	narrowing of joint space (< 3mm)
3:	obliteration of joint or subluxation
4:	bone defect (< 5mm)
5:	bone defect (> 5mm)

Radiologic grades of knees at initial visit and follow-up. Knees injected with intraarticular steroids (top graphs) deteriorated at a rate twice that of non-injected knees (bottom graphs).

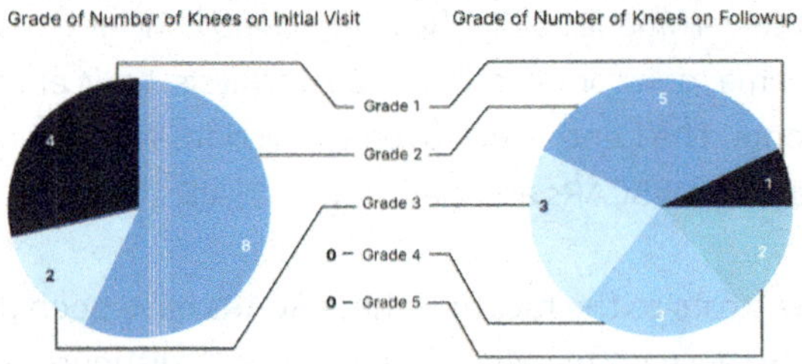

Advancement of Degeneration Rated by Radiological Grade in Corticosteroid-Injected Knees

An illustration of how injected knees degeneration advanced in 11 out of 14 people or 78.6%.

Data from:https://www.airsclinic.com/issue_02_10_deterioration_cartilage.pdf

Corticosteroid injection:
In addition to the use of NSAIDs and regular application of ice to diminish swelling, doctors may rely on the use of a treatment called corticosteroid injection. The primary purpose for corticosteroid injections is to reduce inflammation.

However, unlike NSAIDs and the application of ice, the intention of corticosteroids is to provide a longer lasting anti-inflammatory effect. This treatment has quickly become the standard of care because it does last for a while, typically several weeks to several months of improved pain after a single injection. One could see the benefits of this, except for the negative side effects and the fact that it's not a long-term solution, as I'll explain below.

One other benefit of corticosteroids is that they closely resemble a natural hormone produced in our bodies, called cortisol. We should not view these injections as a natural remedy, even if they do resemble something that is naturally produced in our bodies. In reality, corticosteroids are more often referred to as the condensed term, steroids, which everyone is familiar with, and everyone already knows have side effects.

It is widely known that steroids have a litany of side effects and are often viewed as drugs that should not be considered to treat temporary and acute inflammation conditions. Needless to say, steroids are a divisive treatment option. These injections might not only be dangerous but ineffective and deleterious as well. Dr. Centeno, in his same 2018 study, concluded that corticosteroid injections, "only demonstrate modest clinical benefits without altering disease progression and may increase the rate of cartilage loss."

As we know, osteoarthritis is a result of cartilage loss and anything that has the potential to increase the rate of that cartilage loss should be avoided at all costs. Patients who are aware of these side effects might wonder how these treatments could have been suggested in the first place, and the reality is that while doctors and patients are scrambling for a treatment, anything that relieves pain is seen as a positive until all the side effects are known.

All in all, steroids prohibit the natural function of our immune system to heal and fight infections, a symptom more commonly referred to as immunosuppression. Steroid use makes patients more susceptible to the development and pathogenesis of infections that the immune system would typically fight off. For this reason, it's not recommended for long-term or regular use because it just makes things worse. BUT it's sometimes the only conventional option left. Which again, is why I am working so hard to make genuine stem cell injections for OA, the new conventional medical treatment.

Because steroids are closely tied to cortisol, an artificial supplementation of cortisol to treat OA inflammation can ultimately prohibit the body's natural ability to produce it on its own. Without cortisol or with a low level of cortisol, patients will experience negative effects in multiple systems around the body.

I probably don't need to go into more detail about the side effects and risks of long-term use of steroid injections, but the research coming out in recent years proves that steroid injections are not going to be the future treatment of OA. Even offering them as an option for OA pain on a temporary basis is causing the actual problem of OA to get worse more quickly, so it's just a matter of time before it becomes the wrong course of action for conventional medicine.

Stem cells are really the only viable option in the near future that can tackle both of these issues of improving the condition of the OA affected joint tissues and also relieving pain caused by OA all in one amazing stem cell injection. It's the future and it's already here and available.

Osteopathy, osteopathic manipulative medicine/therapy, OMM/OMT
Osteopathy and osteopathic medicine, with the title of DO, is the same as the MD category of medical title, except that in addition to the entire compendium of medical education you get at MD school, DO physicians learn an extra subject called osteopathic manipulative medicine, which deals with the use of slow and intentional physical manipulations of the body to assist in the medical process. A Doctor of Osteopathic Medicine, DO, is NOT chiropractor.

I know this because I went to DO medical school before I took a leave of absence to open my first big biotech venture.
I also know that what chiropractors learn is vastly different from what a Doctor of Osteopathic Medicine learns. I had friends who were chiropractors, who never learned or heard of many of the techniques I was taught in DO school, which led me to believe that chiropractors are just operating with a whole different mindset of information than a DO, at least from what I can tell with all the providers I've talked to in both categories.

I won't go into all the myriad of different techniques we learned but several of the techniques are designed to reduce inflammation and assist in pain reduction for chronic injuries. Particularly associated with OA of the knee, we learned a technique called the million dollar knee technique.

This million dollar knee technique was a simple maneuver where you have a patient sit on an exam table and hang their legs down. With a bent knee you can see the alignment of the head of the tibia bone with the rest of the knee joint.

Sometimes there is an obvious misalignment upon visible inspection, and here is where the technique works. You can manually apply a mild twisting torque pressure to the head of the tibia to turn it to align with the joint in a proper setting. It's not a permanent fix, but it's just a slow and gradual process of turning that bone to line up and the joint is now able to rest in a better position. This has the effect of reducing the ongoing pressure points within the joint, which were causing all the pain, giving those agitated areas some relief. I'm only presenting what I have seen help on an anecdotal basis because it's just one of the options available. It still has to make sense via the data.

It's only been in the past few years that physicians have begun to evaluate the efficacy of OMT against other forms of treatment for OA. Dr. Åhgren, when studying the efficacy of osteopathy on osteoarthritis, determined that, "despite the nearly 50 non-pharmacological treatment modalities presented today, the research available, at present, omits incorporating osteopathic treatments into research protocols, and fails to contribute with evidence showing if treatments presented enhance the general effectiveness of rehabilitation in decreasing pain and disability in patients subjected to OA." (2021) For this reason, Dr. Åhgren and Skymne examined a series of articles in order to determine whether there was any evidence for osteopathic medicine as a treatment for OA.

They explain that, "seven articles published between 2004 to 2018 were assessed. Three studies aimed to investigate interventions for OA of the knee alone, three involved both the osteoarthritic hip and knee, while one studied OA of the hip exclusively, but the main focus area remained the same, measuring pain severity and physical function. Six of them were randomized controlled trials, while one of them was a longitudinal study."

In the end, doctors Åhgren and Skymne determined that OMT, "can have a beneficial effect in the management of hip and knee OA, however, the presence of osteopathic interventions is as of today very poor in research available and further research is needed to determine the effects of OMT in multimodal clinical practice." OMT needs more time and research before it can conclusively be determined as an effective treatment for osteoarthritis in both the knee and hip joints. Even more consideration will need to be applied when it comes to hand osteoarthritis. However, in terms of safety, OMT osteopathy is generally safe in all applications of treatment and rarely results in any negative side effects when used for these issues and on these particular joint spaces.

So, there is some possible value to some of these OMM procedures for the relief of pain in OA, but again it's just a temporary solution, and when you're in pain almost anything that helps is a win.

Going back to my preference for stem cell treatments for this condition, stem cells are going to be the established standard of care for OA in the future, but all these supportive therapies will likely be useful along the path to getting that stem cell treatment.

Chiropractor

Patients should always consult with their medical physicians before seeking chiropractic adjustments for OA. In general, chiropractic adjustments are not considered an actual treatment for osteoarthritis, but because it's easy and generally considered safe, many doctors will simply suggest that patients try anything that helps as long as it's safe. From cursory discussions on this subject, the relief effect varies widely between patients and relief is temporary. Remember that OA pain is a wear and tear condition. Patients should always consult with their medical physicians before seeking chiropractic adjustments for osteoarthritis.

Diet and exercise (Mediterranean diet)
I want to emphasize that diet and exercise are strong affectors of chronic inflammation, meaning that they can help reduce the overall systemic inflammation that drives your chronic condition, and these can both make it worse if you're not adhering to a good diet. As I mentioned previously, weight can and does have a particularly distinct effect on the progression of osteoarthritis, and weight loss can be a powerful preventative measure.

Without intervention, consistent obesity has a profound effect on the condition of knee and hip joints. This process is clearly explained by Dr. Thomas, who concludes that, "obesity increases strain on weight-bearing joints and, longitudinally, overweight and obese individuals are at considerably higher risk for knee arthroplasty [replacement surgery]. An association of higher BMI with the development of hand OA demonstrates an additional non-biomechanical role of obesity in OA." (2018) Patients could take all the preventative precautions in the world but if they are unable to reduce their weight, the fact remains that their joints will wear down and osteoarthritis will progress and persist.

Dr. Thomas explains that, "Obesity leads to low-grade systemic inflammation and weight reduction can reduce adipose tissue and restore normal secretion patterns. Adipokines could comprise a critical link between obesity and OA. Leptin, an adipokine generally elevated in obesity and produced by white adipose tissue of the infra-patellar fat pad, may underlie this relationship. Leptin is associated with inflammation and cartilage degradation and may be involved in OA pathophysiology at a local and systemic level." (Thomas et al 2018)

Adipokines are signaling molecules associated with fat cells. Adipokines, generally speaking, can either be pro-inflammatory or anti-inflammatory, depending on a patient's level of exercise. Because of the relationship between obesity, adipokines, and osteoarthritis, Dr. Thomas can finally conclude that, "Weight reduction in overweight or obese OA patients reduces joint impact and injurious loading, improves inflammatory adipokine secretion patterns and positively affects metabolic-risk profile." Not only does excess weight contribute to unnecessary strain on the affected joints but pro-inflammatory adipokines that result from a sedentary lifestyle only complicate treatment. With lowered weight comes lower levels of adipose and secreted pro-inflammatory adipokines that exacerbate the condition of osteoarthritis.

I probably don't need to say anything about the Mediterranean diet because there is so much information already available on this subject, but I will say that this is not a "diet" like a weight loss program type of diet. This is a diet as in a lifestyle of eating.

The food variety of the Mediterranean region has a particularly effective result of lowering systemic inflammation and improving overall health and, of course, resulting in natural weight loss to get you to your healthy, normal levels. A nice mix of fruits, nuts, grains, fish, and other healthy items makes up the majority of this diet and it is now the standard of health for medical providers to recommend this diet for nearly everyone.

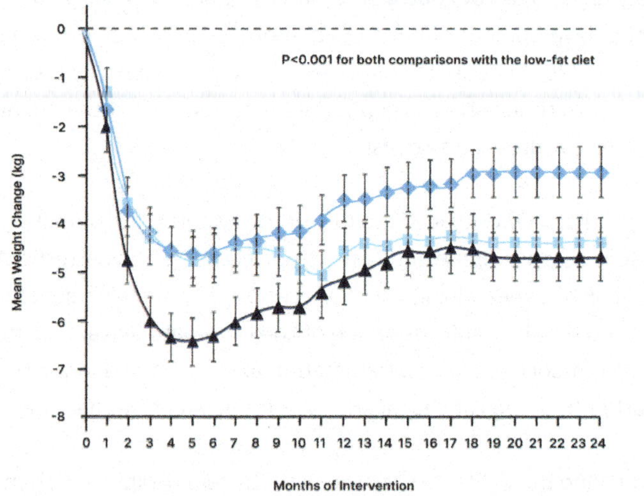

Comparing Low-Carbohydrate, Mediterranean, and Low-Fat Diets in Managing Diabetes

A graph depicting how a Mediterranean diet may be more effective for weight loss and managing diabetes compared to a low-fat diet.

Data from: https://www.nejm.org/doi/full/10.1056/NEJMoa0708681

Embarking on a weight loss journey involves considering different dietary approaches. This includes exploring the effectiveness of low-carbohydrate, Mediterranean, and low-fat diets. Understanding the nuances of these approaches can help individuals make informed choices regarding their weight management goals.

Exercise is also critical, and you'll want to get a great low impact exercise regimen worked out to fit your life and schedule so you can get the benefits of both diet and exercise. I'd also like to throw hydration back into this equation because it's critically important as well.

Surgery (joint replacement surgery for knee and hip)

At a certain point in the progression of OA, there are really no conventional options left, and you'll likely be presented with a knee replacement surgery option. It was discovered in the 1950s and 60s by Dr. John Charnley, who successfully treated the condition by an invasive procedure called arthroplasty. The procedure was relatively successful and continues to be the preferred method for surgical treatment of osteoarthritis.

However, surgical options such as arthroplasty are not considered for patients who have had success maintaining their OA pain through prevention and non-surgical treatment. So, ultimately, this is a last option, and most patients don't want to take this route.

In a medical assessment and survey of advancements in treating OA, Professor K D Brandt of the Indiana University School of Medicine found that "[r]ecommendation of total joint arthroplasty for the patient with OA, however, is tantamount to an acknowledgement of the failure of medical management. The surgical procedure is often performed after the patient has experienced years, or even decades, of pain and disability." (2004)

Patients who have sought treatment for their OA and who are familiar with the "medical management" referred to by Professor Brandt may not have even considered that arthroplasty is only considered for patients who have suffered from its symptoms for years and even decades.

As mentioned by Dr. Brandt, surgery should be (and is often) a last resort for patients because it is the result of medical mismanagement. It is difficult to point the finger when referring to this mismanagement; it is hardly ever entirely the patient's fault nor is it the fault of the physician.

In reality, medical mismanagement refers to a failed process of overall treatment. Ideally, the process begins with an experience of symptoms and on to diagnosis, education, preventative measures, and treatment. Somewhere along the way, one or more of these steps were skipped or ignored.

The unfortunate reality is that diagnosis and early management are often lacking. Arthroplasty and joint replacement surgeries are only considered at the end of the line for treatment options for OA.

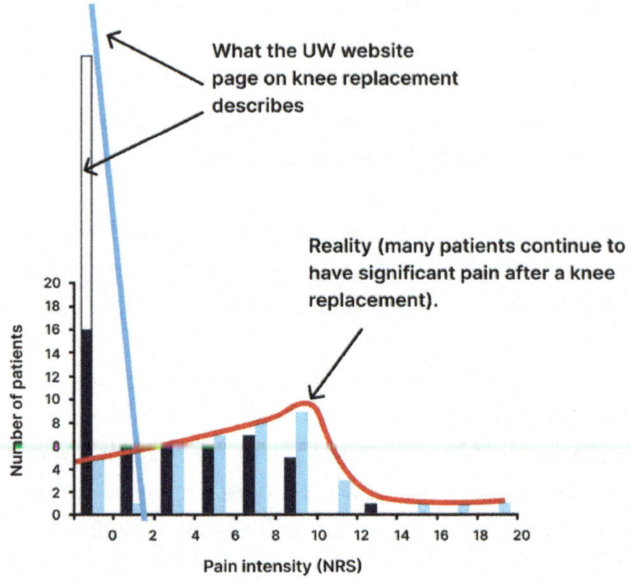

Post-Surgery Pain: Hip vs. Knee Arthroplasty (4-6 Months)

A graph illustrating the comparison between total hip arthroplasty and total knee arthroplasty on the numerical rating scale of worst pain level at 4-6 months after surgery.

Data from: "https://regenexx.com/blog/is-this-the-truth-about-knee-replacement-surgery/

Patients who choose to undergo these arthroplasty events and knee replacement surgeries to relieve their pain are obviously out of safer options. Why would anyone take the risk and the expense if there was any other way to relieve pain and treat OA? After decades of downward spiral and continued OA pain, there just aren't many options left, which is why stem cells for osteoarthritis is the next best option in the lineup to treat OA.

Neurofunctional Pain Management for Osteoarthritis

Neurofunctional Pain Management (NFPM) is another great alternative for chronic pain control that should be considered before undergoing invasive procedures for OA pain relief. The NFPM protocol is comprised of three fundamental components designed to address chronic pain, including OA pain, in a more conservative yet effective approach.

The first component of NFPM is electroanalgesia (EA), a specialized treatment that has the patient undergo high-pulse electrical stimulation. It works by reducing pain signals while simultaneously releasing naturally occurring pain-relieving elements such as neuropeptides, endorphins, enkephalins, and GABA peptides. EA is unique in that it influences the perception of pain by recalibrating the activity of the nervous system's neurons. But most importantly, the reduction of pain signals ultimately creates a positive feedback loop where it also serves to reduce chronic inflammation.

The second component of NFPM is nutritional deficiency specialized IV hydration therapy. This specially tailored IV treatment is adapted to meet each patient's needs, based on a blood test analysis. It aims to correct vital nutritional deficiencies but can also target chronic inflammation as it facilitates the movement of the excess hydrogen ions seen in chronically inflamed tissues. With NFPM protocols, nutritional deficiency hydration IV therapy and EA are used in tandem, which offers a synergistic effect in relieving the chronic systemic inflammation seen in OA patients, potentially providing them with pain relief that endures for months.

The final component is lifestyle counseling, an essential educational program designed to equip patients with the knowledge to make important lifestyle changes while living with a chronic inflammatory disease such as OA. The goal here is to empower individuals to take charge of their own well-being for an overall improved quality of life. And, while NFPM primarily focuses on pain relief, this is where it goes beyond pain management. Rather, it embodies a comprehensive effort to restore health, enhance the quality of patients' lives, and educate individuals in adopting a lifestyle that reduces their reliance on drugs, surgeries, or invasive procedures to hopefully enhance their longevity.

It's likely that many patients would choose NFPM as a first step rather than resorting to surgery, but the key lies in informed decision-making. The guidance and openness of medical professionals play a vital role in introducing patients to effective alternative treatments, avoiding medical mismanagement, and ensuring patients are well-informed of established conservative treatment options.

Chapter 4 – High Dose Stem Cells for Osteoarthritis

Whether it's from a bone marrow aspirate concentration, adipose collection, or an expanded cell culture from birth tissue biologics, stem cell therapy for osteoarthritis is the most promising treatment for OA that is already available in the US and around the world. The ultimate aspect that connects all these is that the concentration of cells needs to be high enough to produce an effective therapeutic outcome.

Currently, the only genuine high dose stem cell treatment for osteoarthritis in the US is via bone marrow aspirate concentrate, BMAC, or adipose collection. This is what I want to talk about first because it's here and now in the US medical market.

I want to say that if you're not eligible for a genuine high dose stem cell treatment using BMAC or adipose, there is always the high dose PRP option that is also a great treatment for osteoarthritis, but this book is about stem cell treatments, and I'll review PRP options in detail in another book.

Bone marrow aspirate concentrate is the official standard source of genuine mesenchymal stem cells in the US medical market. This requires a fairly simple procedure where they aspirate bone marrow from a particular bone in your body, which may vary depending on the individual.

The doctor will likely decide which area is best for collection, and then process the bone marrow to isolate out all the real mesenchymal stem cells and create a concentrated high dose injection of mesenchymal stem cells for injection into the damaged joint.

Remember earlier I discussed how the dose is everything? Well, it's still the case here later in the book: the dose is everything. One of the essential aspects of this process is measuring the quantity and viability of the cells collected and ensuring they are concentrated to an effective therapeutic level.

Much of this has been covered in earlier chapters – the different types of stem cells, how they work to treat conditions, and their increasing prevalence in medicine. Now that you have an increased understanding of stem cells, you might ask what evidence supports stem cell treatment for OA. Relatively speaking, mesenchymal stem cell (MSC) treatment is straightforward.

For the most part, patients who undergo MSC treatment have noticeable pain relief through improved cartilage replacement, which ultimately leads to an enhanced quality of life. However, not all patients will elect to undergo MSC treatment without a deeper understanding of mesenchymal stem cell capability and function.

Mesenchymal stem cells have the capability to repair cartilage affected by osteoarthritis because they are able to target the affected areas, depending on the type of tissue in need of repair. In the case of OA, the tissue in need of repair is the knee, hip, or hand cartilage. Mesenchymal stem cells lead the immune system to reduce inflammation and heal the damaged cartilage.

Dr. Nicholas Tsitsilianos and his associates at the Weill Cornell Department of Rehabilitation Medicine conducted a study evaluating the efficacy of BMAC stem cell injections on the hip. They reported, "[We…] defined response to the treatment as a greater than or equal to 50% reduction in pain compared to their baseline. We also analyzed which patients had at least a 30% reduction in their pain. From this analysis, we found that there was a 42% response rate at 6 months post procedure which increased to a 61% response rate by 12 months. When evaluating 30% reduction in pain, 52% of the cohort by 6 months and 77% of the cohort by 12 months experienced at least a 30% reduction in pain. This demonstrates the time-dependent effect of BMA in improving pain and function in patients with hip OA." (2022)

According to this study, the physicians were able to determine that the longer a patient with hip OA stuck with BMAC stem cell treatment, the greater their reduction in pain.

Cultured Expanded High Dose Stem Cells

As I stated previously, cultured expanded cell therapy refers to taking mesenchymal stem cells and growing them, or replicating them over and over to grow a much larger dose of cells. You can't collect enough natural stem cells in an average bone marrow or adipose collection to treat multiple joints and conditions effectively, so the best way to get more cells is to grow them. The process is called cellular expansion. I've done cellular expansion work many times myself throughout my career in biotech and it's the true future of stem cell therapy. You'll hear the term 'expanded cell therapy,' (or ECT) used to describe this process around the world by the medical and scientific community.

Unfortunately, expanded cell therapy is not permitted in the US and is only available out of the country. Despite it being the future of stem cell therapy, it's still difficult to regulate because there are many variables involved in the process. Some of the most advanced research on expanded stem cells is occurring here in the US, but we can't offer the treatment to patients yet. I'm working actively to get this moving faster here in the US.

Earlier, I described two categories of stem cells: autologous and allogeneic. Autologous means your own cells and allogeneic means a donor's cells. Some companies here in the US may collect bone marrow or adipose cells and offer to culture and expand them for treatment offered out of the country. This has worked so far for many years, but the problem is that you need to have your cells collected, which is invasive in and of itself, then you have to travel to get the treatment. If you're going to have to travel to get expanded cell therapy, you may as well avoid the invasive collection process and use qualified allogeneic stem cell sources that are younger cell lines.

Remember that if you're 70 years old and you collect your own stem cells, you're now using 70-year-old stem cells and the growth capabilities and activity are limited. This doesn't mean those cells aren't useful, but it's obvious that new cell lines have an entire lifespan of activity ahead of them, so the overall understanding of this subject is that younger stem cells are better. If you use allogeneic cell lines, you're using new age 0 stem cells with a full human life cycle of potential growth ahead of them. They are much more active and viable long-term, and this is why the future of stem cell therapy is using cultured expanded birth tissues.

As stated before, we're talking about birth tissues from normal and ethical donation programs where the leftover tissues of regular C-section deliveries can be repurposed into medical therapies instead of being thrown in the medical trash bin. This is from a healthy regular pregnancy where the mother is screened and opts to donate these leftover tissues: the leftover amniotic fluid, placenta, cord tissue, cord blood, and amniotic membrane. All of these materials would simply be disposed of after a C-section, but now we have a way to use it and advance medicine. I'd like to mention here that anyone who has donated tissues to this cause has advanced medical science and I applaud and respect your willingness to do this. Leftover c-section tissue collection is perfectly harmless to the mother and newborn child, so it really is a matter of the mother being willing to allow this donation to happen, so again, I applaud and thank all the women who have volunteered to advance medical science! Thank you!

US regulations need to catch up with medical advancements so we can start doing advanced expanded cell therapy in the US. However, there are qualified medical centers around the world that are offering excellent expanded stem cell therapies.

Contact me directly and I'll refer you to the right places for this! Go to **willbozeman.com** and contact me there. Join my newsletter and other activities to learn all about what's going on in the world of stem cells.

DO NOT shop around the cheapest options in questionable areas of the world. DO NOT use those medical tourism sites to shop, as they will readily let the worst treatment centers buy credibility on their platforms to get patients coming to them, or pay for promotion on those sites even though they are not the best locations for treatment. There are literally no regulations on treatment centers in some areas. ALSO, I know for a fact that in some countries you can simply pay money to bypass regulations to get your medical certifications to set up a stem cell center. Or if you know someone or have a family member in government you can get permission to open a center without much oversight. Be highly careful about where you go internationally for treatment.

I was launching a stem cell treatment center a few years ago, I can't say where for proprietary reasons, when one of the potential partners simply used family connections to bypass the regulations to set up the center. The requirement to do all this basically shifted control of the operation away from our US-based company and into the control of their local operation. At that point I just couldn't be involved because of the extreme risk of not being in control of the medical treatment process, so I exited the operation and have since worked with the top minds in the world on creating the most advanced and reputable stem cell treatment centers. Some of these unscrupulous stem cell centers make wild claims and they also can't document their cell sources and don't have all the right lab processing protocols, or at least they don't release that info to potential patients.

Again, if you want genuine expanded stem cell therapies, contact me and I'll direct you to the best centers around the world who are doing things the right way. There are excellent options, you just have to know where to go.

Because culture expanded stem cells are capable of expanding into other types of cells, this means they are also able to help various parts of the body like the heart or liver. More commonly, culture expanded mesenchymal stem cells are used in the regrowth of tissues and reduction of pain, but are they effective in treating osteoarthritis?

Dr. Ricardo Bastos et al. conducted a study evaluating the efficacy and safety of culture expanded MSCs and platelet rich plasma (PRP) when treating osteoarthritis. These doctors and researchers were able to definitively conclude that, "[a]n intra-articular injection of bone marrow-derived culture-expanded MSCs with or without the [addition] of PRP is effective in improving the function and decreasing symptoms caused by knee OA at 12-month follow-up." (2020) Much like the implementation of BMAC stem cells, the level of efficacy patients experience correlates directly with the length of time they receive the treatment.

The ultimate efficacy of these treatments also depended on the patient's adherence to doctor recommendations. For example, when a patient undergoes BMAC injections in the knee joint, a knee brace is often recommended. This type of mechanical support is used to reduce the stress load on the area treated and improve healing time.

These methods of treatment used in conjunction with the main procedure (being BMAC injection) might seem small, irritating, and unnecessary, but patients would do well to follow these recommendations to ensure the best possible outcomes.

Furthermore, it is promising for Dr. Bastos and his associates to determine that BMAC injection is an effective treatment for OA without an additional application of supplementary treatment. These studies further promote stem cell treatment as an effective and affordable treatment for patient pain.

In addition to treating osteoarthritis pain, patients can have a solid expectation that these stem cells will also repair OA-damaged cartilage. As more and more patients with osteoarthritis find relief through stem cell treatment, there is more conclusive evidence to suggest that it is the next generation of pain treatment and cartilage repair.

Bank Your Own Stem Cells!

Even as an adult you can have your own stem cell cultured, expanded, and banked for future use. Using a simple adipose collection procedure, we can take a small sample of your fat tissue, isolate out the stem cells, and then grow them out in the lab to create dozens of vials of High Dose Stem Cells that are ideal for use down the road. Given the choice would you want to get a stem cell treatment with your own cells or a donor's cells? Most people would pick their own cells.

In the US it's not a standard treatment model yet to use your own cultured expanded stem cells, but you as a person can absolutely have your own cells grown and banked and own them yourself for the future. Once you own your own cells you can do what you want with them later on, so I like to point this out to people who are considering the future treatments that are coming around the corner in the US where it may be OK for people actively get stem cell treatments using their own cells that have been cultured, expanded and banked.

Reach out to me at willbozeman.com, or any of my social media accounts, and I'll connect you with labs that offer this service. Many of the top voices in the industry are already talking about the future acceptance of cultured expanded stem cell therapies in the US and it's going to be an asset for anyone who has their own cells ready to go!

Chapter 5 – Recap and Solutions in the US and Solutions Internationally

Through careful research and review of the scientific data, throughout this book, I have shed light on the complex nature of osteoarthritis and its profound impact on those living with this potentially debilitating condition. It's clear that osteoarthritis is a complex problem that presents a variety of challenges, such as chronic pain, limited movement, and diminishing quality of life for countless individuals all over the world.

Throughout the course of this book, you have learned a lot about the complexities of managing osteoarthritis and have become more educated about the promising alternatives that exist in the realm of stem cell therapies. There is now a glimmer of hope for everyone looking for a way to alleviate the ongoing suffering and avoid the high-risk invasive surgical treatments associated with this condition, benefitting both individuals seeking relief as well as medical professionals searching for efficient treatments with longer-lasting results for patients under their care.

Throughout the chapters of this book, I have provided a thorough look at the current conventional treatment options available for osteoarthritis. This included the commonly prescribed NSAIDs and corticosteroid injections, as well as orthopedic surgical procedures.

While these approaches can offer varying degrees of relief, after this analysis, you are now aware of the limitations associated with these conventional treatments, including their underlying drawbacks and constraints. For instance, NSAIDs offer a temporary option that merely treats the symptoms of osteoarthritis rather than addressing the underlying cause. I have seen this often leave patients dependent on prolonged use of medications with the potential of developing negative side effects as a result. For some people, corticosteroid injections can provide moderate-term comfort; however, in my experience with variable success rates, limited duration of effectiveness, and high likelihood of repeat injections, they too have a number of disadvantages as well as a limited impact on health outcomes.

When seen as the last resort, surgical interventions represent a significant step for patients. It involves substantial recovery and rehabilitation periods as well as the notably heightened risks of complications. By the time this last resort surgical option becomes a possibility, patients have already undergone an exhausting and distressing process through the difficulties associated with osteoarthritis.

I have seen this currently implemented management journey leave patients in disheartening situations in which any hope for effective relief has faded, leaving them naturally hesitant to accept the dangers associated with surgical intervention. This important realization underscores to me the urgency for alternative approaches that offer relief without subjecting individuals to the risks and challenges of invasive procedures.

This exploration into stem cell therapies revealed that bone marrow aspirate concentrate (BMAC), adipose-derived stem cells, and culture-expanded cells all offer unique strengths with distinct advantages in healing and rejuvenating damaged tissues. The essential takeaway from the findings of this regenerative therapy is that the concentration of stem cells is critical to achieving the greatest potential results and optimizing patient health outcomes.

There are some excellent options in the US market for all high dose stem cell therapy using BMAC and/or adipose stem cell therapy for regenerative medicine and osteoarthritis management. Some groups who are standardizing their processes are offering the best options across the nation offering cutting-edge techniques for stem cell therapies and other advanced regenerative therapies. Ultimately, stem cells and regenerative medicine are revolutionizing how osteoarthritis and its numerous challenges are managed.

To reiterate, conventional treatments for osteoarthritis only work for so long, and surgeries and joint replacements may create more problems than they solve. The ideal way to approach OA is with the least invasive options first. Stem cells, PRP, Platelet Lysate, and other injections are truly restructuring the way we treat OA and other degenerative tissue conditions in the US and around the world.

I'd also like to point out that a good physician offering these treatments will likely offer MSK ultrasound guidance and fluoroscopy techniques to guide their injections to the most targeted areas of damage. Traditional medical providers that have a lot of experience don't necessarily need image guidance for injection into large joints, but many of them will acknowledge they prefer to use guidance for surety, because it's good medical practice. Relying on landmarks and going with 'blind' injections isn't ideal, especially if you're paying a lot for the treatment. You want the best possible outcome so use the best techniques to obtain it and element of guesswork. MSK ultrasound provides real-time 3D images of the joint, while fluoroscopy also provides X-ray video that offers a clearer and more comprehensive view. Together, these technologies are excellent and you should look for offices who utilize these image guidance measures.

Where to go in the US for the right treatments?
Visit my website at WillBozeman.com and contact me and I'll send you to the best possible location nearest to you where you can get the best option. I know you may be tempted to just search the internet for this, but I know for a fact that some of the worst players in the field of regenerative medicine have some of the best marketing! So, doing a search in your area will likely bring up several great options, but only a few of them may actually be great and the rest may be either average or inferior even if the cost is lower. REMEMBER, it's the quality of the injection as well as the delivery of the injection that make it work! Just because an office is promoting an inexpensive stem cell of PRP injection doesn't mean it's a good option. If the concentration isn't high enough you won't trigger the regenerative effect and suddenly even that lower priced treatment is WAY overpriced for the benefit you gained. It's much better to pay the extra for a good provider and get the real deal high dose stem cells and high dose PRP!

Can you imagine a future where OA pain doesn't define your day? Or a future where every movement isn't considered for how much pain it will cause? Also, a future where surgery and joint replacements are no longer the default solution, but a rare occurrence for the worst cases?

Where to go for International Stem Cell Treatment Centers?
Connect with me on WillBozeman.com and reach out to me directly and I'll get you to the right locations and the best centers with the most reliable providers and therapies. I don't want to mention any particular center or group here because the international market is always changing and the providers in those centers also changes, so an endorsement in writing can last long after that center loses its status and acceptance as a top level International Stem Cell Treatment Center.

Obviously I've already spent time reviewing all this with you but I want to recap this again. The best options for genuine stem cell therapy and the future of stem cell therapy is using cultured expanded stem cells from perinatal birth tissues. It's the most promising option for wide scale application and convenience. Also, I'm confident that in the coming years this treatment will be refined and standardized and entered into the US market. Also, with scale comes cost and price reduction, allowing for further scale and wider participation. I'm very excited about this. Until then be highly careful about where you go and how you are referred there. Online searches are sometimes dangerous and international medical tourism sites can be bought and paid for by the bad actors. I'm happy to connect you with the best option for the treatment you need by connecting with me on my website willbozeman.com and simply asking me where you should go for treatment. Let's all work together to make stem cell therapy the future of medicine!

Conclusion

By now you have learned quite a bit more than most people know or understand about stem cells and stem cell therapy options inside and outside the US medical market. Also, I hope you know more about some of the other excellent non-stem cell options available here in the US that are still excellent starting points for anyone suffering with osteoarthritis. Remember that a really good PRP is an excellent option as well and that is available here in the US and I can direct you to the right location for that.

Your options in the US are tremendous, so I don't want anyone to think that they can't get some of the best treatments in the world here in the US. The expanded cell therapy market outside the US is much more expensive and difficult to navigate, so I don't like telling people to just go get the latest and greatest from anywhere in the world. I want to make sure those options are vetted so people asking me are going to the right places. Always reach out to me on my personal site to ask about where to go for whatever you're looking for.

My experience in the biotech field and in owning and operating multiple biotech labs and medical practices and various other lab companies has helped me appreciate the complexity of this new era of stem cell therapy. I'm confident in the future of medicine and what we can accomplish. It may be scary to some, but after years of seeing doctors and patients warm up to the new therapy options, and seeing the results, I'm confident that a new wave of acceptance in stem cell therapy will continue to trigger new advancements in the field. I maintain connections across the nation and the world on regenerative medicine to keep my finger on the pulse of what's going on and what is being developed.

If you are uncertain about what you're being told, or what you're reading, the promises of cure and treatment being presented, or even the price of the therapy being offered, reach out to me and I'll help guide you. I can dig into just about any marketing pitch from any practice and see what they are actually offering. I may not be able to advocate for you directly, but I can help guide you on your journey. At the very least I can send you to people who I know will take care of you properly and not simply recite some marketing material to you, or promise you the world and a lifetime of health and happiness for a swipe of your credit card. Let's work together to make regenerative medicine the field it's meant to be and advocate for the good and eliminate the bad. We can do it together!

I look forward to seeing, talking, and connecting with you directly on my personal site **willbozeman.com**.

Thank you so much for reading this book and taking the leap to learn more about this new era of medicine. My last request is that after you have read this book and you've connected with me to guide you on where to go for treatment, give this book to someone else who's suffering from OA. Every little thing we can do for one of us will help all of us!

Sources

Åhgren, K., & Skymne, E. (2021). The Role of Osteopathic Practice in Multimodal Osteoarthritis Care of the Hip or Knee.

Anandacoomarasamy, A., & March, L. (2010) Current Evidence for Osteoarthritis Treatments *Therapeutic Advances in Musculoskeletal Diseases.* 2010 Feb; 2(1): 17–28. doi: 10.1177/1759720X09359889

Barbour KE, Helmick CG, Boring M, Brady TJ. (2017). Vital Signs: Prevalence of Doctor-Diagnosed Arthritis and Arthritis-Attributable Activity Limitation - United States, 2013–2015. *Morb Mortal Wkly Rep.*

Bastos, R., Mathias, M., Andrade, R., Amaral, R. J., Schott, V., Balduino, A., ... & Espregueira-Mendes, J. (2020). Intra-articular injection of culture-expanded mesenchymal stem cells with or without addition of platelet-rich plasma is effective in decreasing pain and symptoms in knee osteoarthritis: a controlled, double-blind clinical trial. *Knee Surgery, Sports Traumatology, Arthroscopy,* 28, 1989-1999.

Brandt, K.D. (2004). Non-surgical treatment of osteoarthritis: a half century of "advances." *Annals of the Rheumatic Diseases.* 63:117-122.

Centeno, C., Sheinkop, M., Dodson, E. et al. (2018). A specific protocol of autologous bone marrow concentrate and platelet products versus exercise therapy for symptomatic knee osteoarthritis: a randomized controlled trial with 2 year follow-up. *J Transl Med* 16, 355.

Hunter, David J et al. (2019). *The Lancet,* Volume 393, Issue 10182, 1745-1759.

Magni,A., Agostoni, P., Bonezzi, C., Massazza, G., Menè, P., Savarino, V., &Fornasari, D. (2021) *Management of Osteoarthritis: Expert Opinion on NSAIDs Pain Ther.* 2021 Dec 10(2): 783-808

Mylan New Zealand Ltd. (2009). *Noflam Data Sheet* 2 February.

New Zealand Government (2012) NSAIDs can SCAR (*Severe Cutaneous Adverse Reaction*) MEDSAFE New Zealand Medicines and Medical Devices Safety Authority https://www.medsafe.govt.nz/profs/PUArticles/NSAIDScanSCARJune2012.htm retrieved August 2023

NHIS (2013-2015) National Health Interview Survey
Novartis New Zealand Ltd. (2010). *Diclofenac Sandoz Data Sheet* 18 November.

Osteoarthritis Action Alliance (OAAA), OA PREVALENCE AND BURDEN https://oaaction.unc.edu/oa-module/oa-prevalence-and-burden/ Retrieved August 2023

Reyes, C., Leyland, K.M., Peat, G., Cooper, C., Arden, N.K. and Prieto-Alhambra, D. (2016). Association Between Overweight and Obesity and Risk of Clinically Diagnosed Knee, Hip, and Hand Osteoarthritis: A Population-Based Cohort Study. Arthritis & Rheumatology, 68: 1869-1875.

Thomas, S., Browne, H., Mobasheri, A., & Rayman, M. P. (2018). What is the evidence for a role for diet and nutrition in osteoarthritis? *Rheumatology,* 57(suppl_4), iv61-iv74.

Tsitsilianos, N., Shirazi, Z., Lu, J., & Singh, J. R. (2022). Bone marrow aspirate injection for osteoarthritis of the hip; A pilot study. *Interventional Pain Medicine,* 1(4), 100163.

Made in the USA
Monee, IL
03 November 2026

67378710R00046